Surface Marking Of

KEYNOTES

(A Revolutionary Way of Learning Materia Medica)

DR. AZAD RAI
D.I.Hom. (London), D.H.M.S. (Medalist), B.H.M.S. (Pb.)

Asstt.Prof. : Deptt. of Materia Medica, Sri Guru Nanak Dev
　　　　　　 Homeopathic Medical College & Hospital, Ludhiana.
Author　　 : Scholar's Manual of Homeopathic Materia Medica
Editor　　　: Allen's Keynotes - 10th Edition

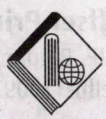

B. Jain Publishers (P) Ltd.
AN ISO 9001 : 2000 CERTIFIED COMPANY
NEW DELHI, INDIA

Surface Marking Of
KEYNOTES

First Edition: 2006

All rights are reserved. No part of this book may be reproduced, stored in a retrieval system or transmitted, in any form or by any means, mechanical, photocopying, recording or otherwise, without any prior written permission of the publishers.

© Copyright with the Publishers.

Price: Rs. 175.00

Published by **Kuldeep Jain** *for*

B. Jain Publishers (P) Ltd.
AN ISO 9001 : 2000 CERTIFIED COMPANY
1921, Street No. 10, Chuna Mandi, Paharganj,
New Delhi-110 055 (INDIA).
Phone: 91-11-23580800, 23583100, 23581300, 23581100
Fax: 91-11-23580471, **Email:** bjain@vsnl.com
Website: www.bjainbooks.com

Printed in India by:
J.J. Offset Printers
522, FIE, Patpar Ganj,
Delhi-110092.

ISBN : 81-8056-723-0
Book Code : BR-5929

DEDICATED
to my
Lovely Kids
Keshav *and* Vinayak

PREFACE

'Surface Marking of Keynotes' is a new and very interesting method of studying materia medica. From the time of Dr. Hahnemann, different types of materia medicas have been developed in homeopathy to make the materia medica easy and comprehensive.

The idea of writing this book is to present the materia medica in a simple, comprehensive and practical form. This is one of its first attempt to create materia medica in such a form. Every possible attempt has been made to present the individualistic features of every drug to make the study interesting and within easy grasp.

In this book three different colour dots (red, blue, green) are marked on the body surface to denote the location and gradation of symptoms covered by that particular drug. In this way we can easily frame a picture or get an impression in our mind about that drug regarding which part of body is most affected by it and in which intensity it is affected.

It is not possible to mark all symptoms on body surface because there are symptoms like those of mind and physical generals e.g. hemorrhages, pains, rheumatism, anemia, marasmus, bones, glands, thirst, sweat, sleep, prostration, dropsy, skin etc., which pertains to whole body. But these symptoms are integral part of the body and drug pathogenesis, so they are marked separately in a little box along with body sketch.

Drug symptoms are written opposite to the body sketch on one side of the book. Only most striking, characteristic, peculiar, uncommon, very important and clinical symptoms are taken in each drug.

Symptoms are arranged preferably according to their clinical importance under three grades and not in an anatomical presentation. It helps to simplify and strengthen our selection of a particular drug with its relative importance by gradation. It makes the study of materia medica extremely interesting and also lowers the burden of memorizing the full pathogenesity of each drug.

As scope of improvement in any new project is always there, I shall be glad to receive any constructive suggestions for the betterment of this book.

I wish to extend my heartfelt gratitude to God, the creature of world, who blessed me with this ability to create a new method of studying materia medica.

I am greteful to my grandmother, Late Smt. Krishnavati Rai, whose warmth, love, affection, encouragement and blessings shall ever stay as a treasure in my remembrance. Words perhaps fail to express the deep sense of gratitude I owe to my grandmother.

I am grateful to my father Sh. Khushbakhat Rai and mother Smt. Ranjana Rai, who gave me inspiration to work hard all through my life.

I am happy to record the co-operation and help I have received from my wife Dr. Geetika Rai and my brother Mr. Aman Rai, whose zeal and devotion have made my task easier.

Finally I also wish to record my thanks to Sh. Kuldeep Jain of B. Jain Publishers (P) Ltd., New Delhi, for his support, guidance and encouragement.

13th January, 2006   **Dr. Azad Rai**
Lohri   B-XXIII, 486, St. No. Zero
                                           Janak Puri, Ludhiana, Punjab
                                                      Mob.: 09876850406

ABOUT THE AUTHOR

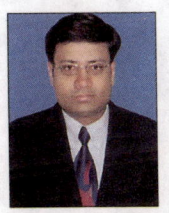Born on 15th August, 1974, Dr. Azad Rai did D.H.M.S. with merit, B.H.M.S. (Graded Degree) and is pursuing M.D. (Hom.) in Homeopathic Materia Medica from Sri Guru Nanak Dev Homeopathic Medical College & Hospital, Ludhiana. Presently he is also teaching as Assistant Professor of Materia Medica in the same college. He is examiner for Baba Farid University of Health Sciences, Faridkot. Dr. Rai is also engaged in Private Practice for the last 10 years. He has contributed many articles in various journals, magazines and national dailies. He has edited 10th edition of "Allen's Keynotes" published in 2004. "Scholar's Manual of Homeopathic Materia Medica" authored by him is very useful for homeopathic students and practitioners.

CONTENTS

Preface iii
About the Author vii
Abrotanum 3
Aceticum acidum 5
Aconitum napellus 7
Actaea racemosa 9
Aesculus hippocastanum 11
Aethusa cynapium 13
Agaricus muscarius 15
Agnus castus 17
Allium cepa 19
Aloe socotrina 21
Alumina 23
Ambra grisea 25
Ammonium carbonicum 27
Ammonium muriaticum 29
Anacardium orientale 31
Antimonium crudum 33
Antimonium tartaricum 35
Apis mellifica 37
Apocynum cannabinum 39
Argentum metallicum 41
Argentum nitricum 43
Arnica montana 45
Arsenicum album 47
Arsenicum iodatum 49
Arum triphyllum 51
Aurum metallicum 53
Baptisia tinctoria 55
Baryta carbonica 57
Belladonna 59
Berberis vulgaris 61
Bismuthum 63
Borax 65
Bovista 67
Bromium 69
Bryonia alba 71
Cactus grandiflorus 73
Calcarea arsenica 75
Calcarea carbonica 77
Calcarea fluorica 79
Calcarea phosphorica 81
Calcarea sulphurica 83
Calendula 85
Camphora 87
Cantharides 89
Carbo vegetabilis 91
Causticum 93
Chamomilla 95
Chelidonium majus 97
Cina 99
Cinchona officinalis 101
Colchicum autumnale 103
Colocynthis 105

ix

SURFACE MARKING OF KEYNOTES

Conium maculatum 107	Mercurius 157
Digitalis purpurea 109	Mercurius corrosivus 159
Drosera rotundifolia 111	Natrum carbonicum 161
Dulcamara 113	Natrum muriaticum 163
Euphrasia 115	Natrum phosphoricum 165
Ferrum metallicum 117	Natrum sulphuricum 167
Ferrum phosphoricum 119	Nitric acid 169
Gelsemium sempervirens 121	Nux moschata 171
Graphites 123	Nux vomica 173
Helleborus niger 125	Opium 175
Hepar sulphuris 127	Petroleum 177
Hyoscyamus niger 129	Phosphorus 179
Ignatia amara 131	Phytolacca decandra 181
Ipecacuanha 133	Platinum metallicum 183
Kali bichromicum 135	Podophyllum 185
Kali bromatum 137	Pulsatilla 187
Kali carbonicum 139	Rhus toxicodendron 189
Kali muriaticum 141	Secale cornutum 191
Kali phosphoricum 143	Sepia 193
Kali sulphuricum 145	Silicea 195
Kreosotum 147	Spongia tosta 197
Lachesis 149	Sulphur 199
Ledum palustre 151	Thuja occidentalis 201
Lycopodium clavatum 153	Veratrum album 203
Magnesia phosphorica 155	

Surface Marking of KEYNOTES

ABROTANUM

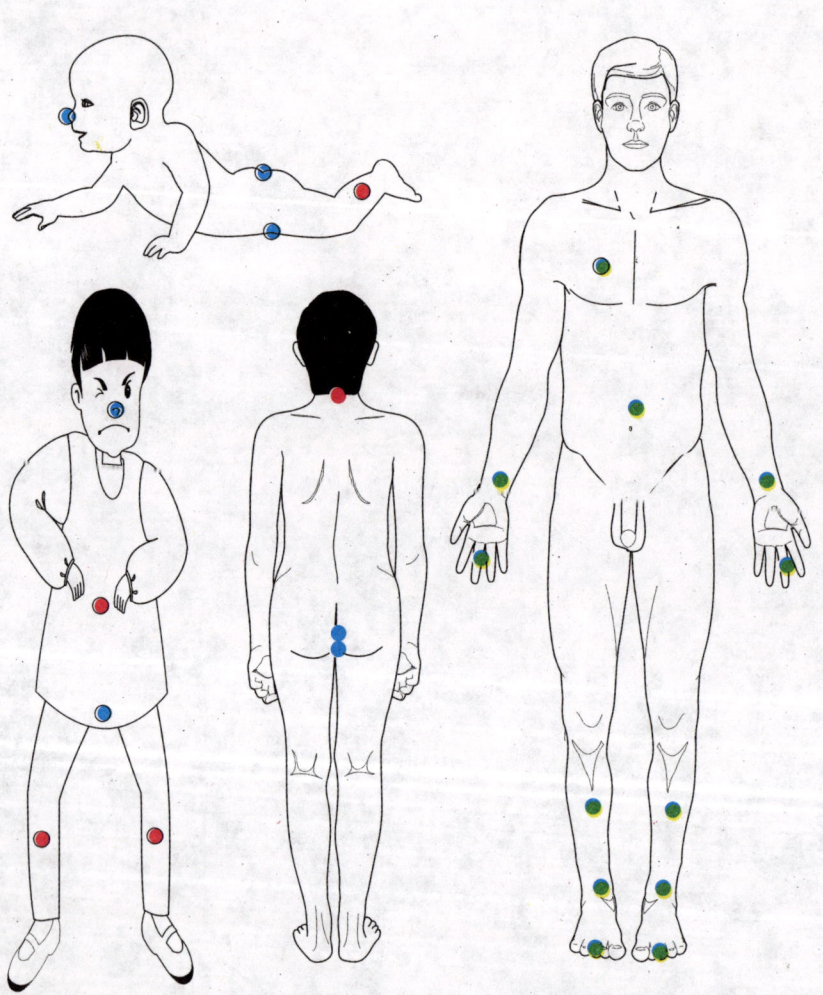

ABROTANUM

Southernwood
Compositae

- Child is ill-natured, irritable, cross and violent.
- Marasmus of children with marked emaciation, especially of legs.
- In Marasmus, head weak, cannot hold it up.
- Ravenous hunger; losing flesh while eating well.

- Alternate constipation and diarrhea; lienteria.
- Rheumatism from suddenly - checked diarrhea or other secretions.
- Rheumatism alternates with hemorrhoids, with dysentery.
- Newborn or children especially boys, who suffer from hydrocele or epistaxis.

- Painful contractions of the limbs from cramps or following colic.
- Gout: Joints stiff, swollen with pricking sensation; wrists and ankle-joints painful and inflamed.
- In pleurisy, when a pressing sensation remains in affected side impending respiration.
- Itching chilblains.

SURFACE MARKING OF KEYNOTES

ACETICUM ACIDUM

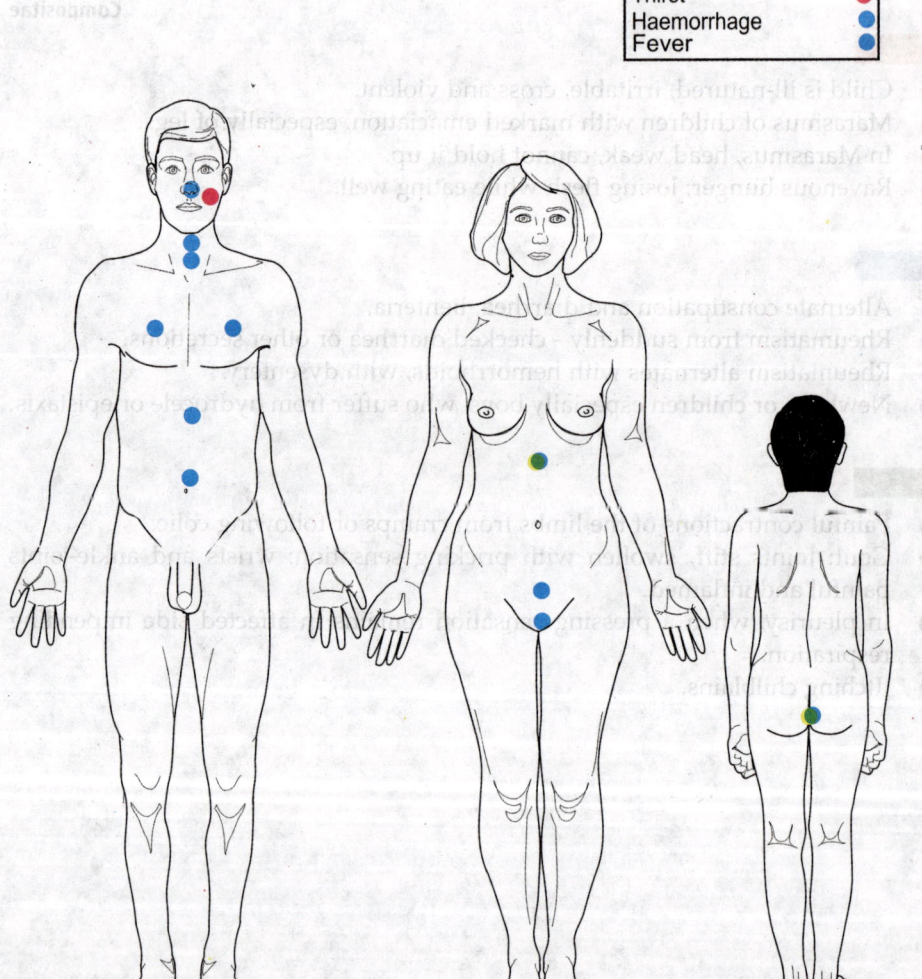

Marasmus ●
Dropsy ●
Thirst ●
Haemorrhage ●
Fever ●

4 A

ACETICUM ACIDUM

Glacial Acetic Acid
CH_3COOH

- Adapted to pale, lean persons with lax, flabby muscles; face pale, waxy.
- Marasmus and other wasting diseases of children.
- General anasarca, dropsical affections, ascites.
- Thirst: intense, burning, insatiable even for large quantities in dropsy, diabetes, chronic diarrhea; but no thirst in fever.

- Hemorrhage: From every mucus outlet, nose, throat, lungs, stomach, bowels, uterus; menorrhagia, vicarious; traumatic epistaxis.
- True croup, hissing respiration, cough with the inhalation; last stages.
- Hectic fever, skin dry and hot; red spot on left cheek and drenching night sweats.

- Sour belching and vomiting of pregnancy, burning water brash and profuse salivation, day and night.
- Diarrhea: Copious, exhausting, great thirst; in dropsy, typhus, phthisis; with night sweats.

SURFACE MARKING OF KEYNOTES

ACONITUM NAPELLUS

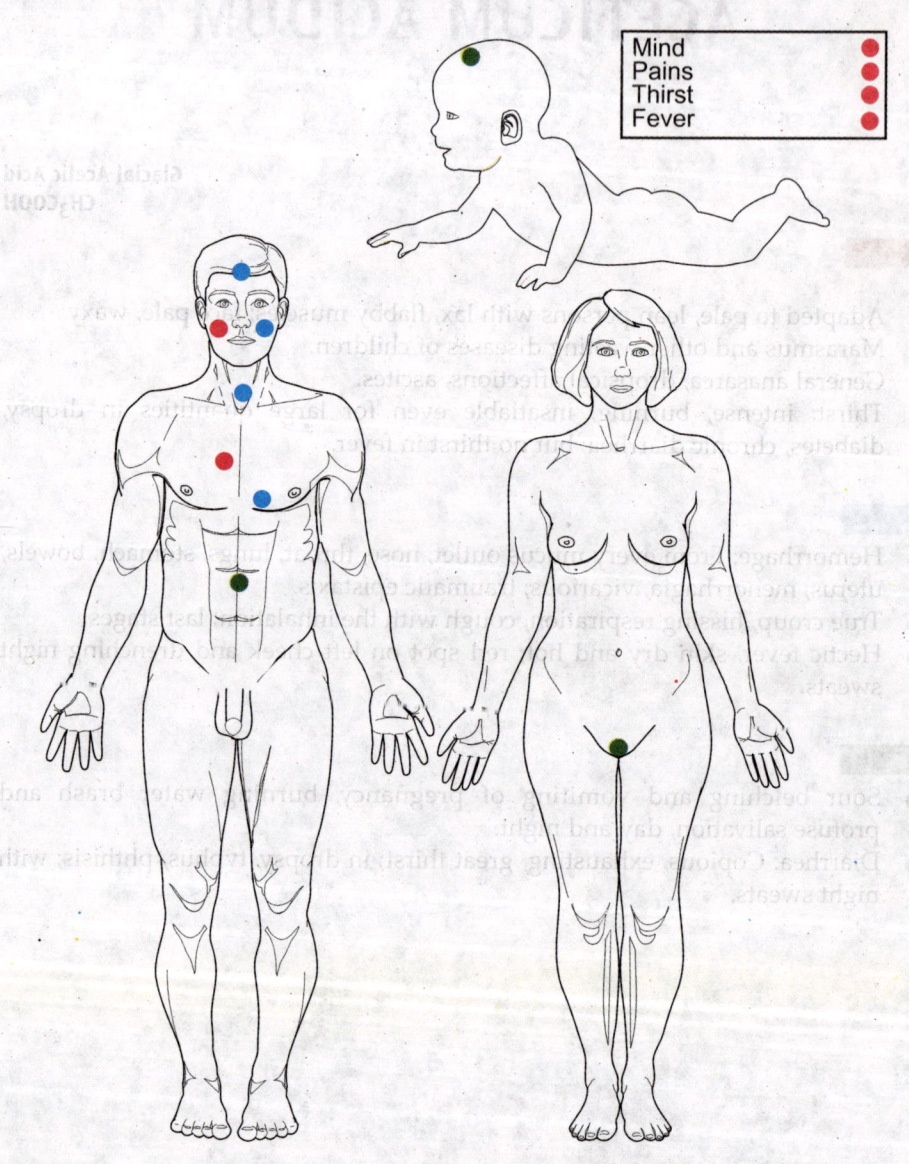

6 A

ACONITUM NAPELLUS

Monkshood
Ranunculaceae

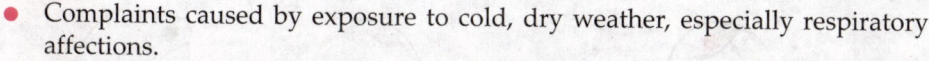

- Complaints caused by exposure to cold, dry weather, especially respiratory affections.
- Mental anxiety, restlessness, worry, fear accompanies the most trivial ailment.
- Pains: are intolerable, they drive him crazy; at night.
- For the congestive stage of inflammation before localization takes place.
- Burning thirst for large quantities of cold water.
- Fever: Skin dry and hot; face red, or pale and red alternately; becomes intolerable towards evening and on going to sleep.

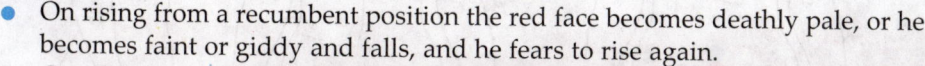

- On rising from a recumbent position the red face becomes deathly pale, or he becomes faint or giddy and falls, and he fears to rise again.
- Cough, croup, dry, hoarse, suffocating; loud, rough, croaking; hard, rising, whistling; on expiration; from dry, cold winds or drafts of air.
- Palpitation, with anxiety, fainting and tingling in fingers, pain down left arm.

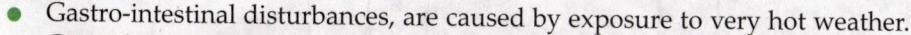

- Gastro-intestinal disturbances, are caused by exposure to very hot weather.
- Convulsions: of teething children; heat, jerks and twitches of single muscles; child gnaws its fist, frets and screams; high fever.
- Suppression of menses from fright or cold, in plethoric young girls.

SURFACE MARKING OF KEYNOTES

ACTAEA RACEMOSA

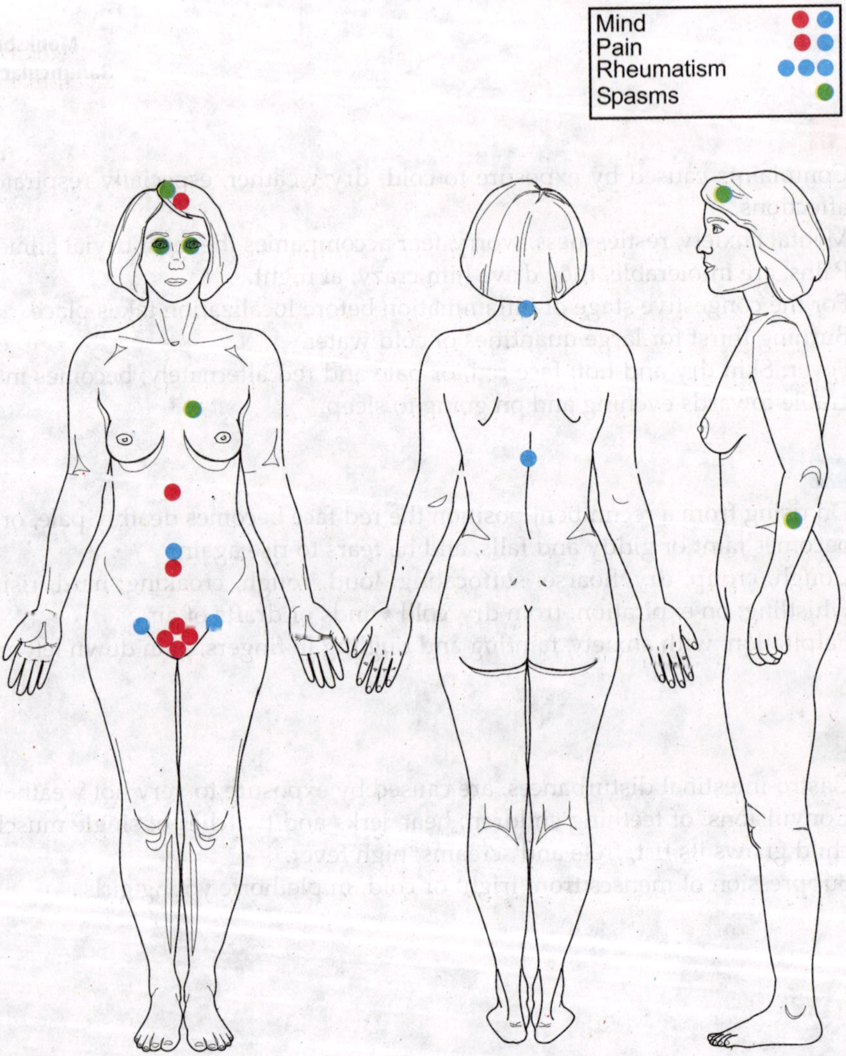

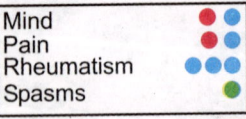

Mind	🔴
Pain	🔴🔴
Rheumatism	🔵🔵🔵
Spasms	🟢

8 A

ACTAEA RACEMOSA

Black Cohosh
Ranunculaceae

- Menses: Irregular, exhausting; delayed or suppressed by mental emotion, from cold, from fever, with chorea, hysteria or mania; increase of mental symptoms during menses; more flow, more pain.
- Pregnancy; nausea; sleeplessness; false labor - like pains; sharp pains across abdomen; abortion at third month.
- During labor: "Shivers" in first stage; convulsions, from nervous excitement; rigid os; pains severe, spasmodic, tedious, < by least noise.
- Given before the term; it renders labor easier, cures sickness of pregnancy, prevents the after pains.
- It ensured living births, in women who have previously borne only dead children without any discoverable cause.

- Mania following disappearance of neuralgia.
- Excessive muscular soreness, after dancing, skating, or other violent muscular exertion.
- Rheumatic pains in muscles of neck and back.
- Rheumatic pains in muscles of neck and back.
- Sharp, lancinating electric - like pains in various parts, sympathetic with ovarian or uterine irritation.

- Spasms: hysterical or epileptic; reflex from uterine disease, worse during menses; chorea < left side.
- Heart troubles from reflex symptoms of uterus or ovaries. Heart's action ceases suddenly; impending suffocation; palpitation from least motion.
- Ciliary neuralgia; pains in globes, extending to vertex, < slightest motion, going up stairs, > pressure, lying down.

SURFACE MARKING OF KEYNOTES

AESCULUS HIPPOCASTANUM

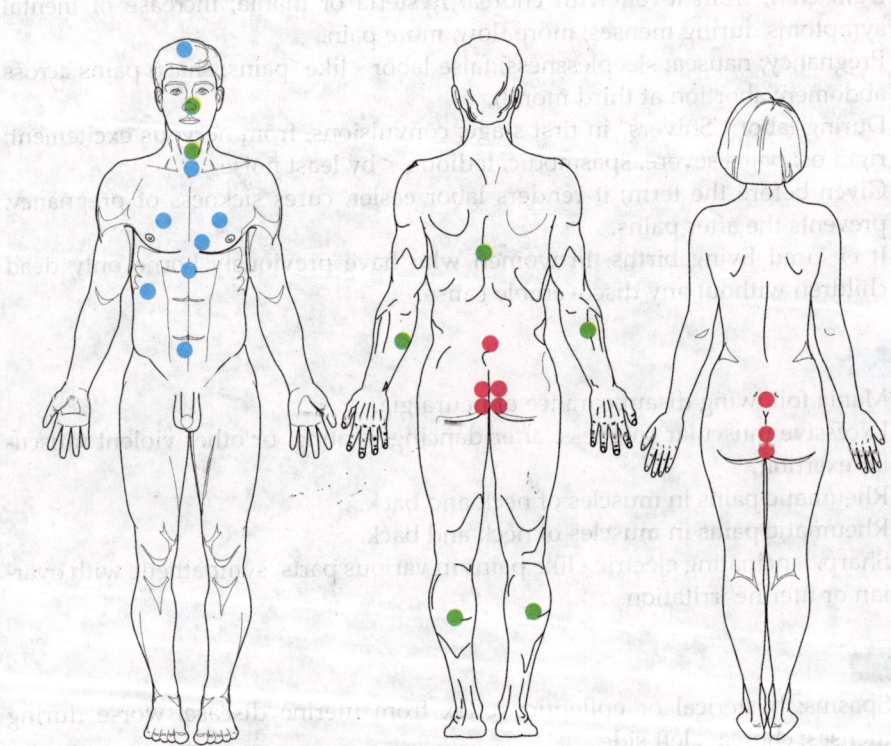

AESCULUS HIPPOCASTANUM

Horse Chestnut
Sapindaceae

- Constipation: hard, dry stool, difficult to pass; with dryness and heat of rectum.
- Rectum feels as if full of small sticks.
- Stool followed by fullness of rectum and intense pain in anus for hours.
- Hemorrhoids blind, painful, burning, purplish, rarely bleeding.
- Severe dull backache in lumbo-sacral articulation; more or less constant.
- Back "gives out": during pregnancy, prolapsus uteri, leucorrhoea; when walking or stooping; must sit or lie down.

- Venous congestion, especially portal and hemorrhoidal.
- Fullness in various parts, as from an undue amount of blood, liver, heart, lungs, brain, stomach, abdomen, pelvis, skin.
- Mucous membranes of mouth, nose, throat, rectum are swollen, burn, feel dry and raw.

- Follicular pharyngitis: Violent burning, dry, raw sensation in throat.
- Coryza: thin, watery, burning; rawness and sensitive to inhaled cold air.
- Paralytic feeling in arms, legs and spine.

SURFACE MARKING OF KEYNOTES

AETHUSA CYNAPIUM

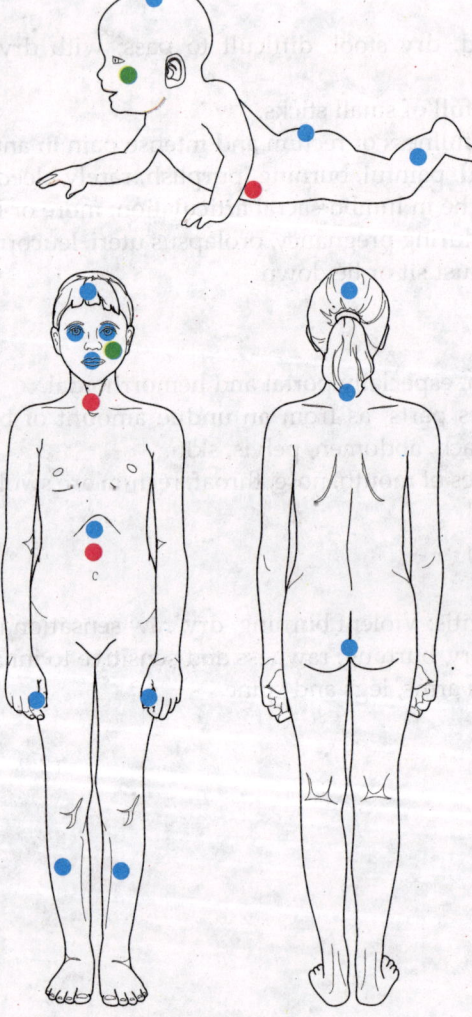

Thirstless	●
Prostration	●●
Spasm	●
Mind	●●

12 A

AETHUSA CYNAPIUM

**Fool's Parsley
Umbelliferae**

- Indigestion of teething children; violent, sudden vomiting of a frothy, milk-white substance; or yellow fluid, followed by curdled milk and cheesy matter.
- Can not bear milk in any form; it is vomited in large curds as soon as taken; then weakness causes drowsiness.
- Complete absence of thirst.

- Great weakness: children cannot stand; unable to hold up the head.
- Prostration with sleepiness; after vomiting, after stool, after spasm.
- Epileptic spasms, with clenched thumbs, red face, eyes turned downwards, pupils fixed and dilated; foam at the mouth, jaws locked; pulse small, hard, quick.

- Idiocy in children; incapacity to think; confused.
- An expression of great anxiety and pain, with a drawn condition and well-marked linea nasalia.

SURFACE MARKING OF KEYNOTES

AGARICUS MUSCARIUS

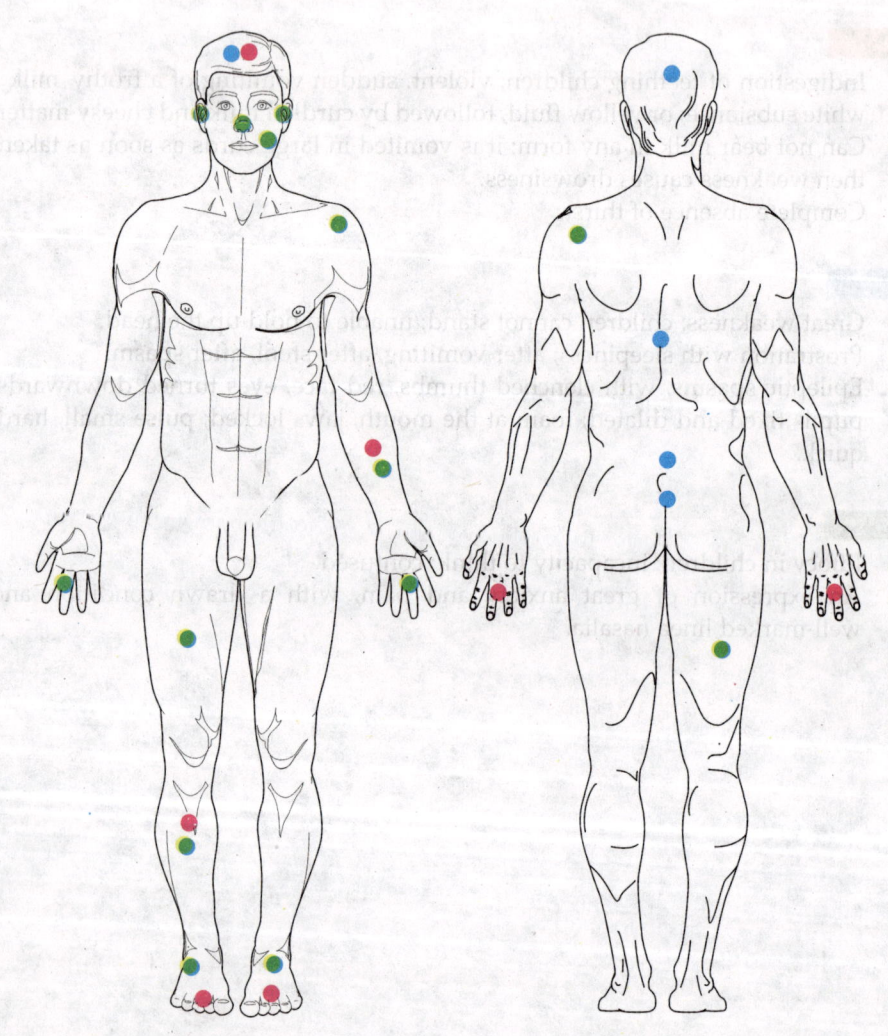

AGARICUS MUSCARIUS

Toadstool
Fungi

- Involuntary movements while awake, cease during sleep.
- Chorea, from simple motion and jerks of single muscle to dancing of whole body; trembling of whole body.
- Uncertainty in walking, stumbling gait, stumbles over everything in the way.
- Epilepsy from suppressed eruptions.
- Chilblains, that itch and burn intolerably; frostbite and all consequences of exposure to cold.

- Drunkards, especially for their headaches; bad effects after a debauch.
- Pain; sore aching in lumbar and sacral regions; during exertion in the day time; while sitting.
- Every motion, every turn of body, causes pain in spine, < morning. Single vertebra sensitive to touch.
- Spinal irritation due to sexual excesses.

- Burning, itching, redness of various parts; ears, nose, face, hands and feet; parts red, swollen, hot.
- Sensation as if ice touched or ice-cold needles were piercing the skin; as from hot needles.
- Complaints appear diagonally; upper left and lower right side.

SURFACE MARKING OF KEYNOTES

AGNUS CASTUS

Mind ●

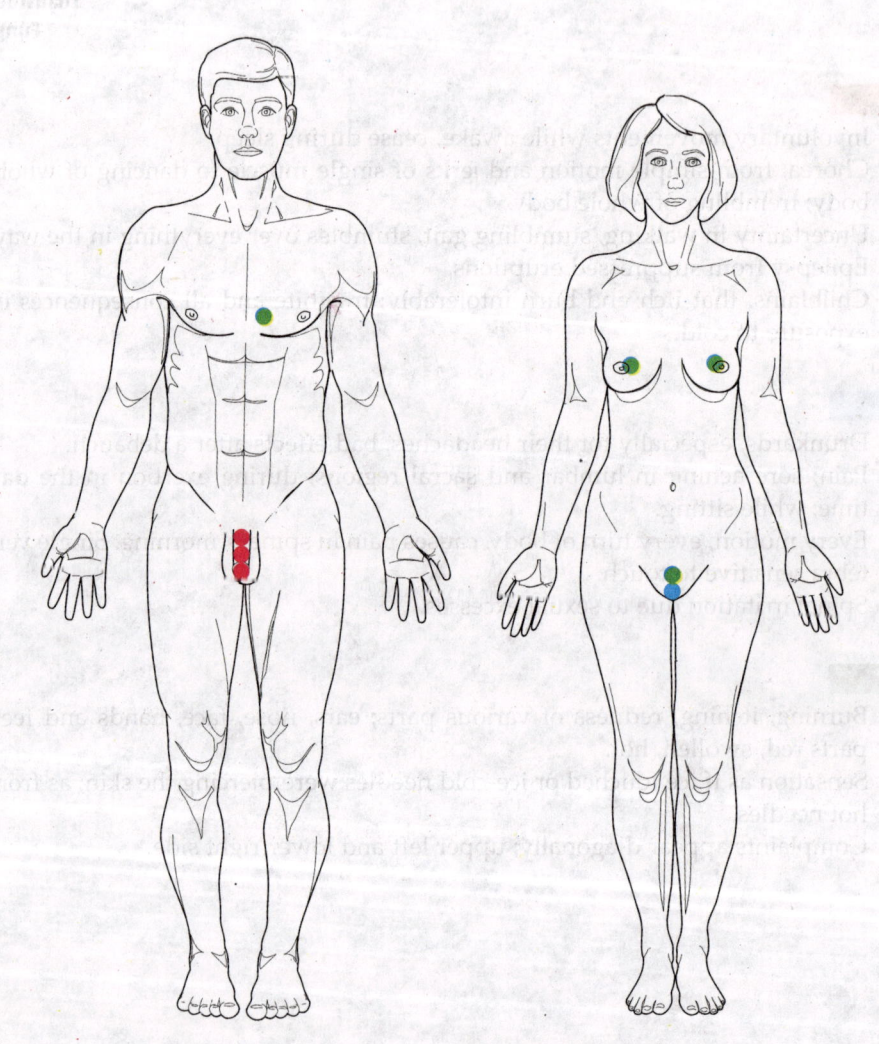

16 A

AGNUS CASTUS

Chaste tree
Verbenaceae

- Premature old age: melancholy, apathy, mental distraction, self contempt; arising in young persons from abuse of the sexual powers; from seminal losses.
- Complete impotence: relaxation, flaccidity, coldness of genitalia. No sexual power or desire.
- Impotence, after frequent attacks of gonorrhea.

- Absent-minded, reduced power of insight.
- Unmarried persons suffering from nervous debility.
- Leucorrhoea; transparent, but staining linen yellow; passes imperceptibly from the very relaxed parts.

- Agalactia, with sadness.
- Sterility; with suppression of menses and no sexual desire.
- Sprains and strains.
- Tachycardia caused by tobacco in neurotic young men.

SURFACE MARKING OF KEYNOTES

ALLIUM CEPA

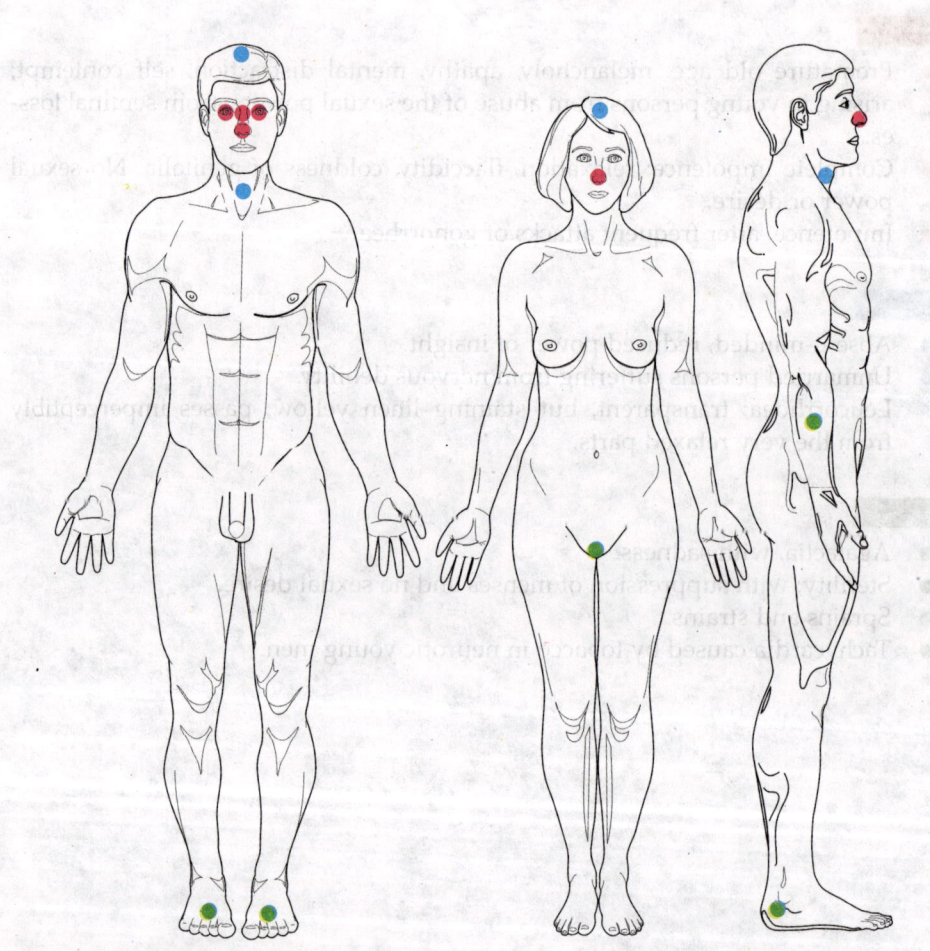

18 A

ALLIUM CEPA

Onion
Liliaceae

- Coryza; profuse, watery and acrid nasal discharge, with profuse, bland lachrymation.
- Spring coryza; after damp northeasterly winds.
- Hay fever; in August every year; violent sneezing on rising from bed.

- Catarrhal dull headache, with coryza; < in evening, > in open air; < on returning to a warm room.
- Headache ceases during menses; returns when flow disappears.
- Catarrhal laryngitis; cough compels patient to grasp the larynx; seems as if cough would tear it.

- Traumatic chronic neuritis; neuralgia of stump after amputation; burning and stinging pains.
- Neuralgic pains like a long thread following injuries to the nerves or amputation or other surgical operations.
- Sore and raw spots or ulcers on feet, from friction; skin is rubbed off by the shoes especially on the heels.
- Phlebitis, puerperal; after forceps delivery.

SURFACE MARKING OF KEYNOTES

ALOE SOCOTRINA

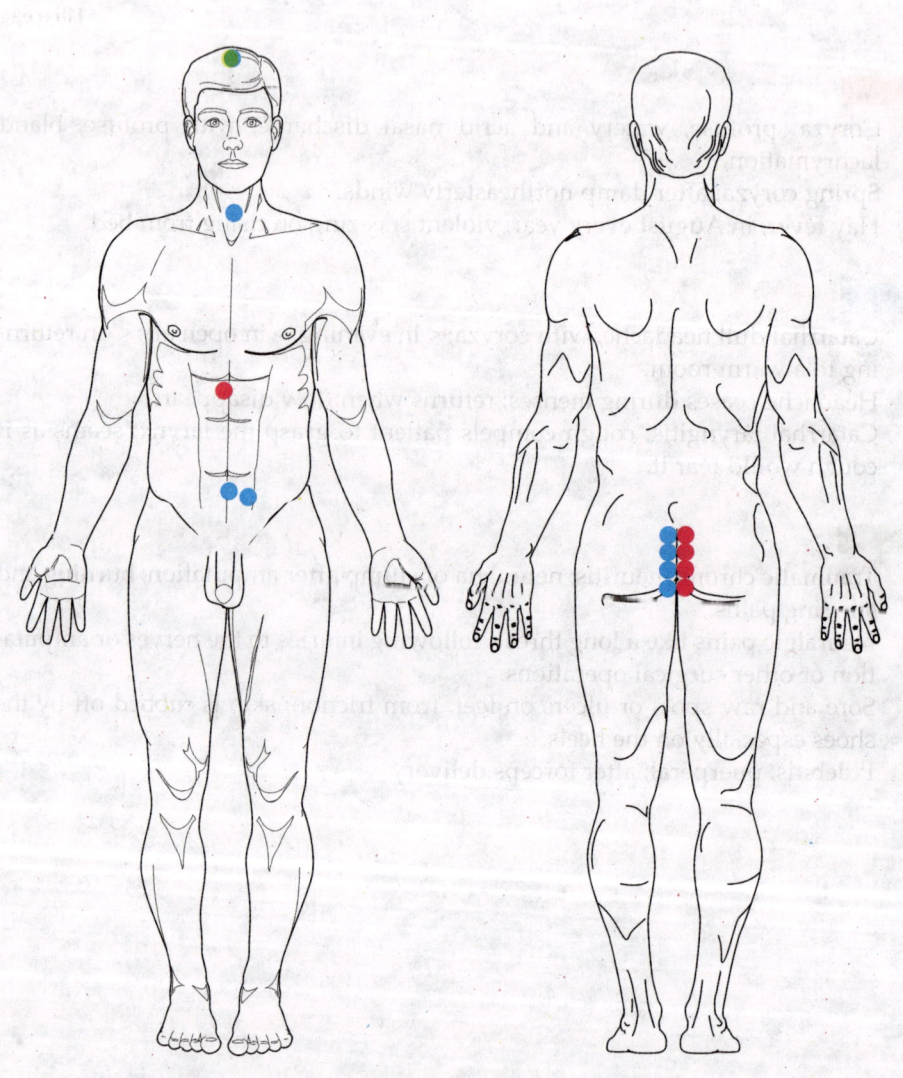

ALOE SOCOTRINA

Socotrine Aloes
Liliaceae

- Diarrhea; after eating oysters; in hot season, or of beer drinkers.
- Diarrhea; has to hurry to closet immediately after eating and drinking; with want of confidence in sphincter ani; driving out of bed early in the morning.
- Hungry during diarrhoea.
- When passing flatus, sensation as if stool would pass with it.
- Flatus offensive, burning, copious; much flatus with small stool.

- Production of mucus in jelly-like lumps from throat or rectum.
- Hemorrhoids: blue, like a bunch of grapes, constant bearing down in rectum; bleeding, sore, tender, hot, relieved by cold water; itching and burning in anus, preventing sleep.
- Colic; excruciating, before and during stool; all pains cease after stool, leaving profuse sweating and extreme weakness; attacks preceded by obstinate constipation.
- Before stool; rumbling, violent sudden urging, heaviness in rectum.
- During stool, tenesmus and much flatus.
- After stool, faintness.

- Dissatisfied and angry about himself or his complaints, especially when constipated.
- Headaches: are worse from heat, better from cold applications; alternating with lumbago; after insufficient stool.

SURFACE MARKING OF KEYNOTES

ALUMINA

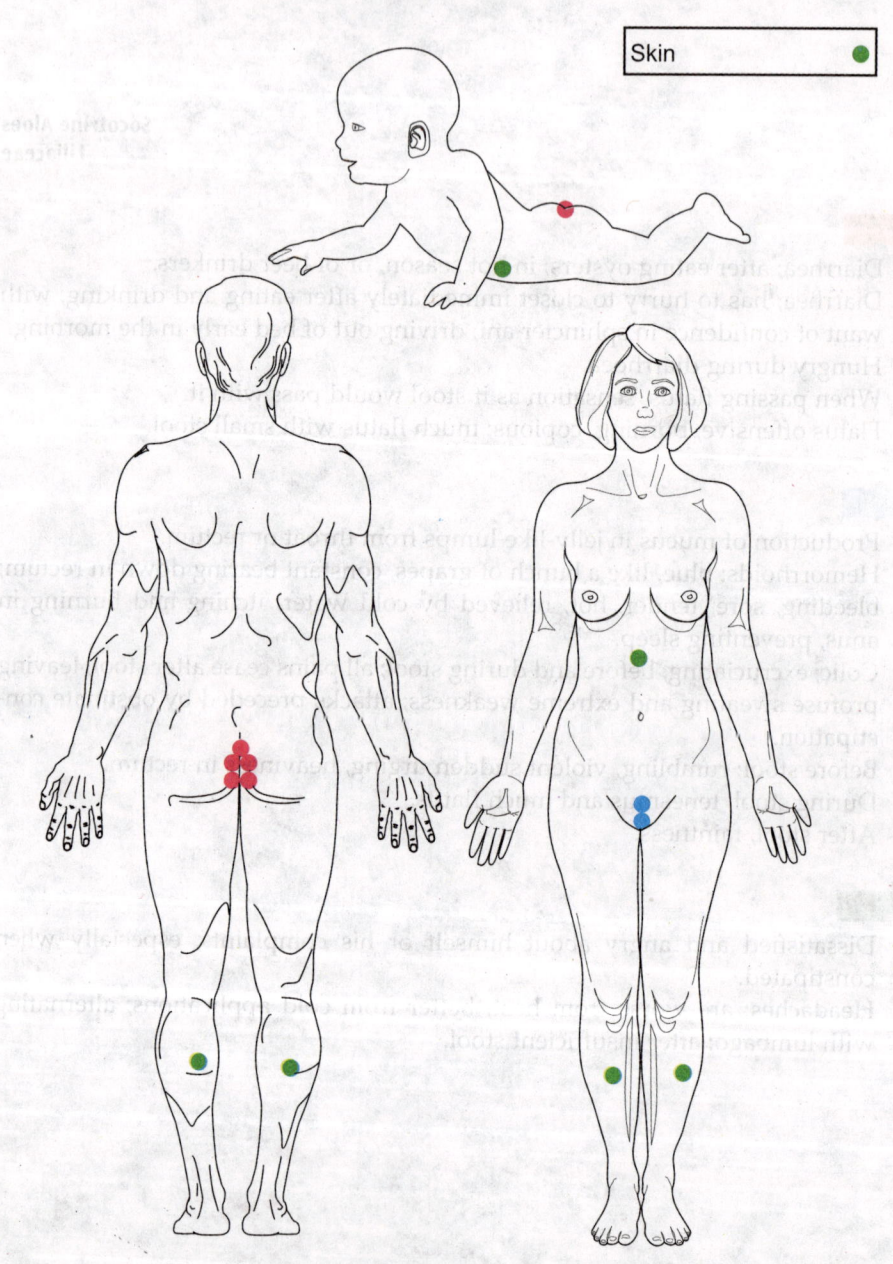

ALUMINA

Pure clay
Al(OH)₃

🟥
- Constipation: no desire for and no ability to pass stool until there is a large accumulation.
- Inactivity of rectum, even soft stool requires great straining, must grasp the seat of closet tightly.
- Can only pass stool when standing.
- Stool hard, knotty, like laurel berries, covered with mucus; or soft, clayey, adhering to parts.
- Constipation: of nursing children, from artificial food; bottle-fed babies; of old people; of pregnancy, from inactive rectum.

🟦
- Menses, too early, short, scanty, pale followed by great physical and mental exhaustion.
- Leucorrhoea: acrid and profuse, running down to the heels; worse during the day time; > by cold bathing.

🟩
- Abnormal craving for indigestible things.
- Aversion to potato, to meat, which disagrees.
- Inability to walk, except with the eyes open, and in the daytime; tottering and falling when closing eyes.
- Dry, tettery, itching eruption, worse in winter, full and new moon; intolerable, itching of whole body when getting warm in bed; scratches until bleeds, then becomes painful.

A 23

SURFACE MARKING OF KEYNOTES

AMBRA GRISEA

Mind

Pure clay
Al(OH)₃

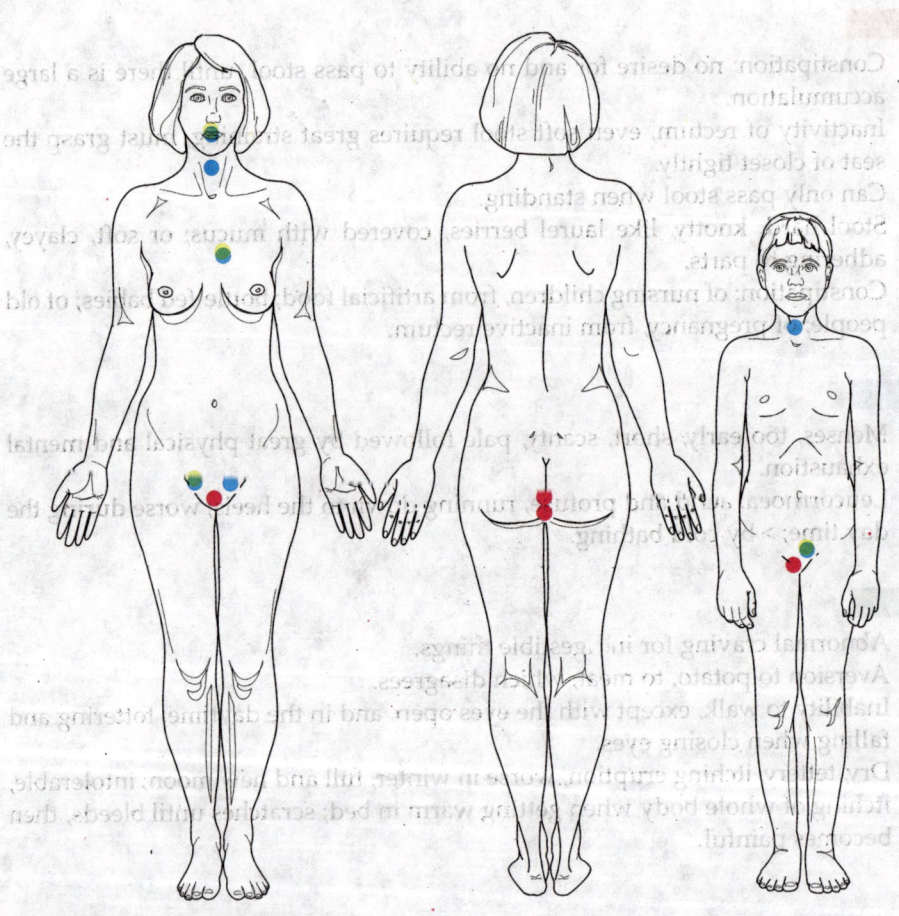

24 A

AMBRA GRISEA

Ambergris
A Nosode

- For children especially young modern society girls who are excitable, nervous and weak; hysterical subjects; nervous affections of old people; thin scrawny women.
- The presence of others, even the nurse, is unbearable during stool and urination.
- Frequent ineffectual urging for stool.
- Constipation, during pregnancy and after delivery.
- Leucorrhoea: thick, bluish-white mucus, especially or only at night.

- Discharge of blood between periods, at every little accident—a long walk, after every hard stool, etc.
- Violent cough in spasmodic paroxysms, with eructations and hoarseness; < music, in presence of many people, talking and reading aloud, lifting weight; evening without, morning with bluish white expectoration.

- Itching of pudendum, with soreness and swelling.
- Ranula with fetid breath.
- Shock due to business failure or deaths one after another in the family.
- Slight or unusual things aggravates the breathing, the heart or start the menses etc.

SURFACE MARKING OF KEYNOTES

AMMONIUM CARBONICUM

Haemorrhage ●

26 A

AMMONIUM CARBONICUM

Smelling Salts
$2NH_4O_3CO_2$

🔴
- Stopping of nose, mostly at night, with long lasting coryza, must breathe through the mouth.
- Snuffles of children.
- Nose bleed: When washing the face and hands in the morning; after eating or on waking.
- Diphtheria or scarlatina when the nose is stopped up.
- Tonsils and neck glands are enlarged; tendency to gangrenous ulceration of tonsils.

🔵
- Cholera like symptoms at the commencement of menses.
- Menses: too early, profuse, clotted, black with griping colic and hard difficult stools; acrid, makes the thighs sore; copious at night and when sitting; with toothache, sadness; with fatigue especially of thighs, yawning and chilliness.
- Hemorrhagic diathesis.

🟢
- One of the best remedies in emphysema.
- Dyspnoea with palpitation worse by exertion or on ascending even a few steps; worse in a warm room.
- Loses breath when falling asleep, must awaken to get breath.
- Cough every morning from 3 to 4 a.m.
- Malignant scarlatina with deep sleep.

SURFACE MARKING OF KEYNOTES

AMMONIUM MURIATICUM

| Obesity | ● |

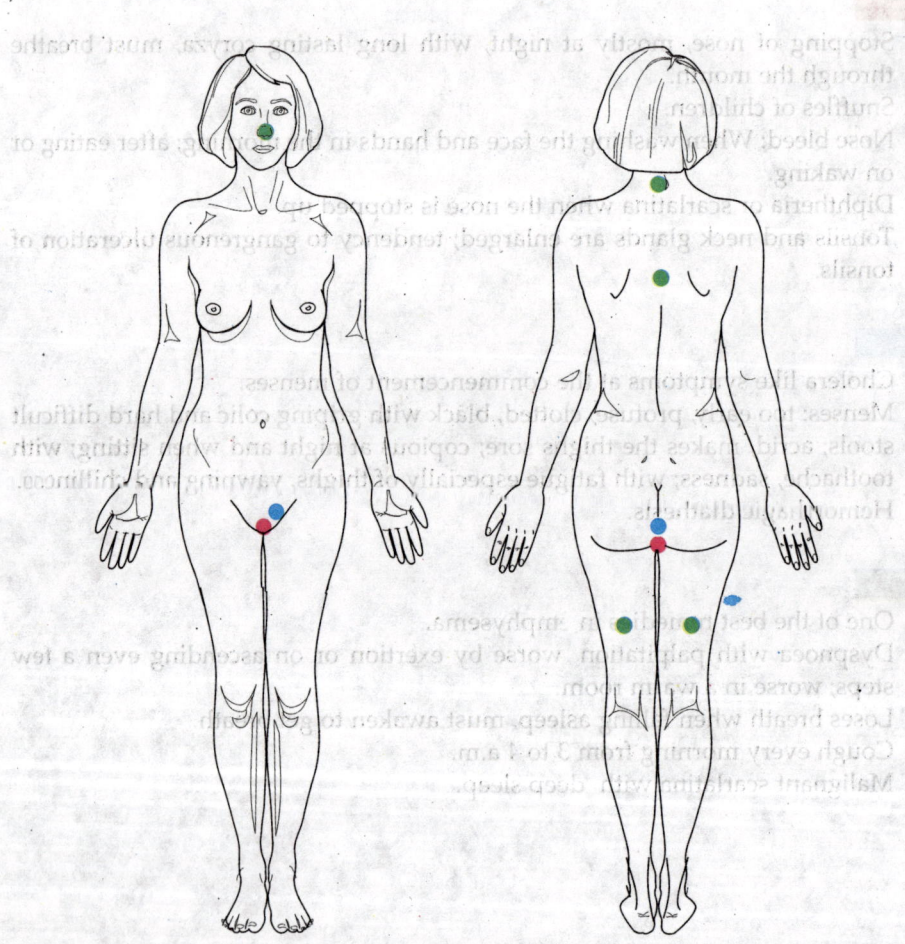

28 A

AMMONIUM MURIATICUM

Sal Ammoniac
NH₄Cl

- Especially adapted to those who are fat and sluggish; or body large and fat, but legs too thin.
- Hard crumbling stools require great effort in expulsion; changing colour and consistency, no two stools alike.
- During menses; diarrhea and vomiting, bloody discharge from the bowels; neuralgic pains in the feet; flow more profuse at night.

- Leucorrhoea: like white of egg, preceded by griping pain about the navel; brown, slimy, painless, after every urination.
- Hemorrhoids: sore and smarting; with burning and stinging in the rectum for hours after stool especially after suppressed leucorrhoea.

- Watery, acrid coryza, corroding the lip.
- Hamstrings feel painfully short when walking; tension in joints as from shortening of the muscles.
- Swelled cervical glands.
- Sore sprain or icy coldness between scapulae, not relieved by warmth.

SURFACE MARKING OF KEYNOTES

ANACARDIUM ORIENTALE

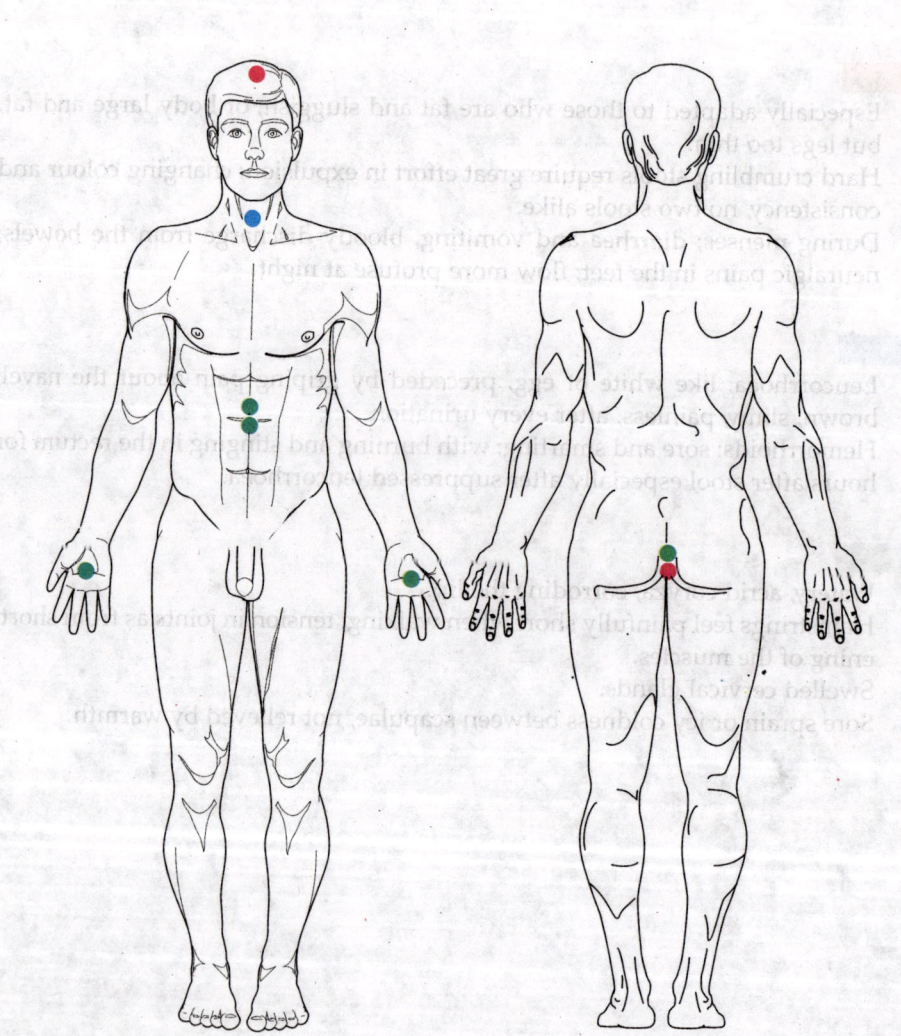

ANACARDIUM ORIENTALE

Marking Nut
Anacardiaceae

- Sudden loss of memory; everything seems to be in a dream, patient is greatly troubled about his forget-fulness.
- Irresistible desire to curse and swear.
- Feels as though he had two wills.
- Headache: relieved entirely when eating; when lying down in bed at night, and when about falling asleep; worse during motion and work.
- Great desire for stool, but with the effort the desire passes away without evacuation; rectum seems powerless, paralyzed, with sensation as if plugged up.

- Weakness of all the senses.
- Sensation; as of a hoop or band around a part; as of a plug in inner parts.
- Swallows food and drink hastily; symptoms disappear while eating.

- Hypochondriac, with hemorrhoids and constipation.
- Empty feeling in stomach.
- Gastric pains > by eating, but < again after 2 to 3 hours.
- Warts on palms of hands.
- Dermatitis; itching < scratching.

SURFACE MARKING OF KEYNOTES

ANTIMONIUM CRUDUM

Mind ● ● ●

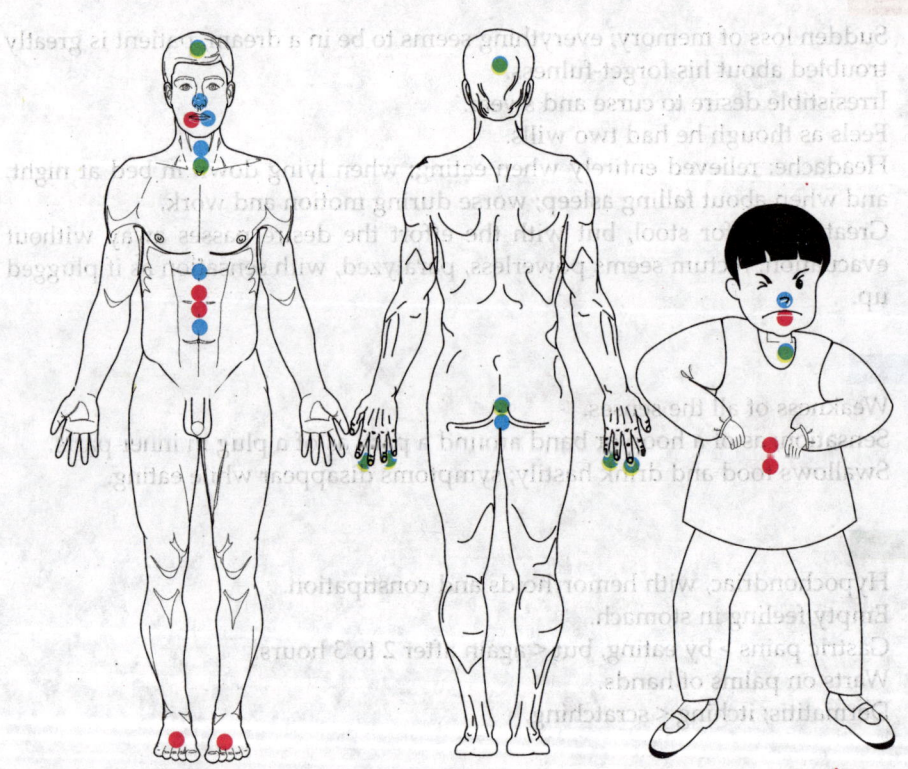

Marking Nut
Anacardiaceae

ANTIMONIUM CRUDUM

Sulphide of Antimony
Sb_2S_3

- For children and young people inclined to grow fat.
- Child is fretful, peevish, cannot bear to be touched or looked at.
- Great sadness, with weeping.
- Sentimental mood in the moonlight.
- Cannot bear the heat of sun; exhausted in warm weather.
- Aversion to cold bathing.
- A thick milky-white coating on the tongue.
- Gastric complaints from over-eating.
- Stomach weak, digestion easily disturbed.
- Large horny corns on soles of feet.

- Nostrils and labial commissures sore, cracked and crusty.
- Mucus in large quantities from posterior nares by hawking.
- Gastric and intestinal affections; from bread, pastry, acids especially vinegar, sour or bad wine, over heating, hot weather; after cold bathing.
- Mucus from anus, ichorous, oozing, staining yellow; mucus piles.

- Headache: after river bathing; from taking cold; alcoholic drinks; deranged digestion, acids; fat, fruit; suppressed eruption.
- Loss of voice from becoming over-heated.
- Whooping-cough < by over heating, in a warm room.
- Alternate diarrhea and constipation.
- Fingernails do not grow rapidly; crushed nails grow in splits like warts with horny spots.

A 33

SURFACE MARKING OF KEYNOTES

ANTIMONIUM TARTARICUM

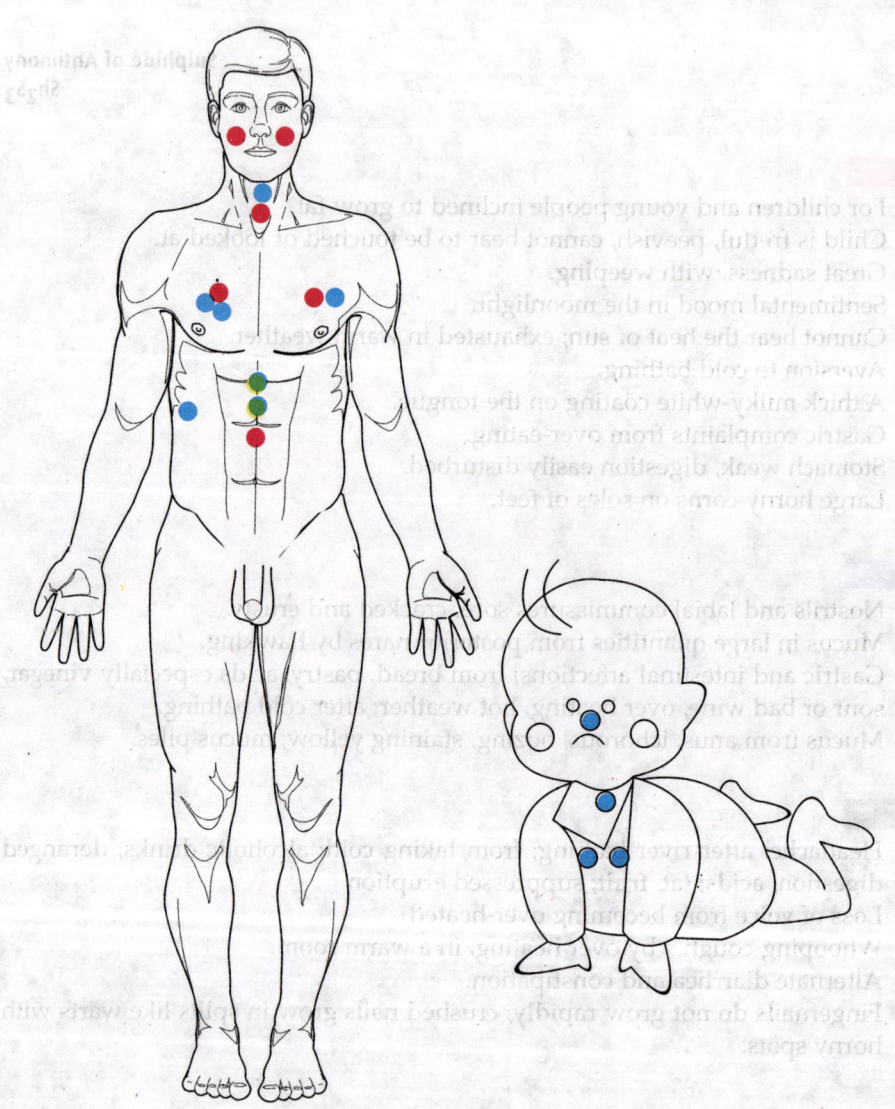

34 A

ANTIMONIUM TARTARICUM

Tartar Emetic
$2[K(SbO)C_4H_4O_6]H_2O$

- Adapted to torpid, phlegmatic persons; the hydrogenoid constitution.
- Great sleepiness or irresistible inclination to sleep, with nearly all complaints.
- Extraordinary craving for apples.
- Face cold, blue, pale, covered with cold sweat.
- When the patient coughs there appears to be a large collection of mucus in the bronchi; it seems as if much would be expectorated, but nothing comes up.

- Asphyxia; mechanical, as apparent death from drowning; from mucus in bronchi; from impending paralysis of lungs; from foreign bodies in larynx or trachea; with drowsiness and coma.
- Child at birth pale, breathless, gasping; asphyxia neonatorum. Relieves the "death-rattle".
- Spasmodic motion of alae-nasi.
- Jaundice with pneumonia, especially of right lung.

- Vomiting in any position except lying on right side; until he faints.
- Vomiting forcible, followed by drowsiness and prostration.
- Pustular eruption leaving a bluish-red mark.
- Thick eruptions like pocks.

A 35

SURFACE MARKING OF KEYNOTES

APIS MELLIFICA

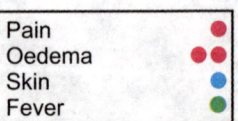

36 A

APIS MELLIFICA

Poison of the Honey Bee
Apium Virus

- Pain: burning, stinging, sore; suddenly migrating from one part to another.
- Affects serous membranes of heart, brain, pleura etc., produces inflammation with effusion.
- Oedema; of hands, feet, and various parts with shiny, red-rosy colour.
- Bag-like, puffy swelling under the eyes.
- Dropsy without thirst.

- Affects right side; enlargement or dropsy of right ovary; right testicle.
- Incontinence of urine, with great irritation of the parts; can scarcely retain the urine a moment, and when passed scalds severely.
- Urine frequent, painful, scanty, bloody.
- Bad effects of acute exanthema imperfectly developed or suppressed; measles, scarlatina, urticaria.
- Tumors or open cancer of mammae.

- Constipation: sensation in abdomen as if something tight would break if much effort were used.
- Diarrhea: of drunkards; in eruptive disease, especially if eruption be suppressed; involuntary from every motion, as though anus was wide open.
- Intermittent fever; chill 3 p.m. with thirst, always; < warm room and from external heat; heat of one part with coldness of another.

SURFACE MARKING OF KEYNOTES

APOCYNUM CANNABINUM

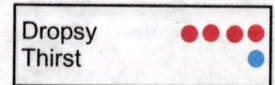

Dropsy
Thirst

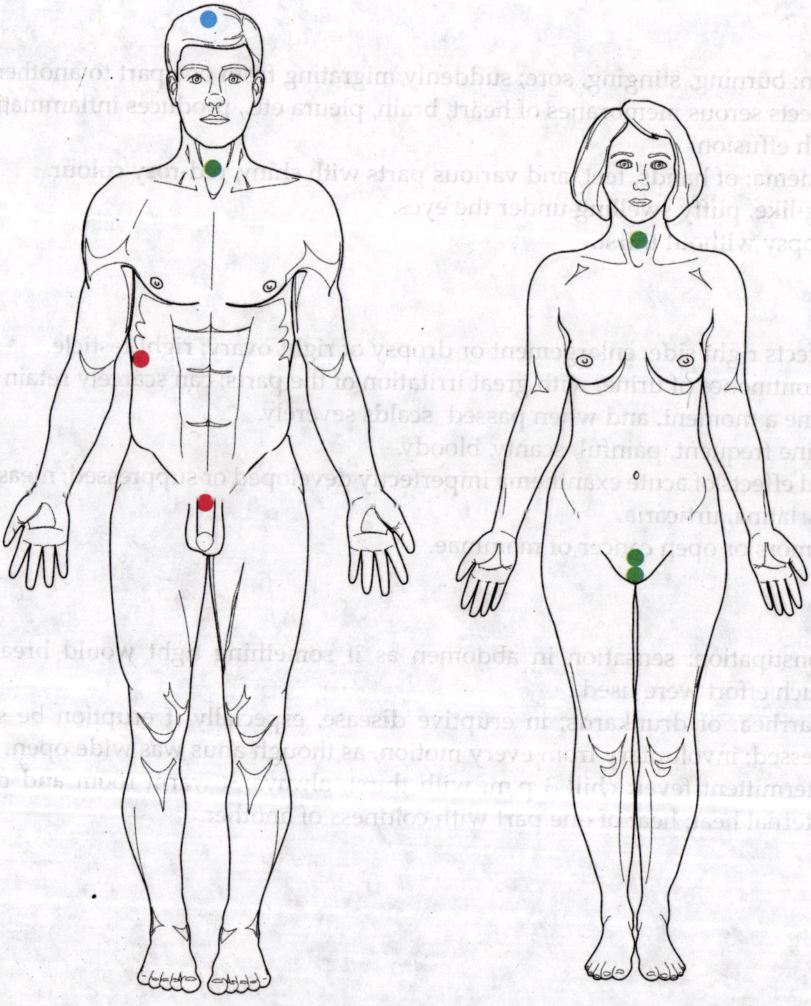

38 A

APOCYNUM CANNABINUM

Indian Hemp
Apocynaceae

- Dropsy of serous membranes; acute, inflammatory; with thirst.
- Dropsy with or without organic disease.
- Dropsy; after typhus, typhoid, scarlatina, cirrhosis, hemorrhage; after abuse of quinine.
- Swelling of every part of body, with scanty urine and sweat.

- Acute hydrocephalus, with open sutures, projecting forehead, stupor, loss of vision and with automatic motion of one arm and leg.
- Thirst, but water disagrees, is vomited at once in dropsy.

- Amenorrhoea in young girls, with bloating of abdomen and extremities.
- Metrorrhagia; continued or paroxysmal flow; fluid or clotted; at climaxis.
- Cough; short and dry, or deep and loose; during pregnancy.

SURFACE MARKING OF KEYNOTES

ARGENTUM METALLICUM

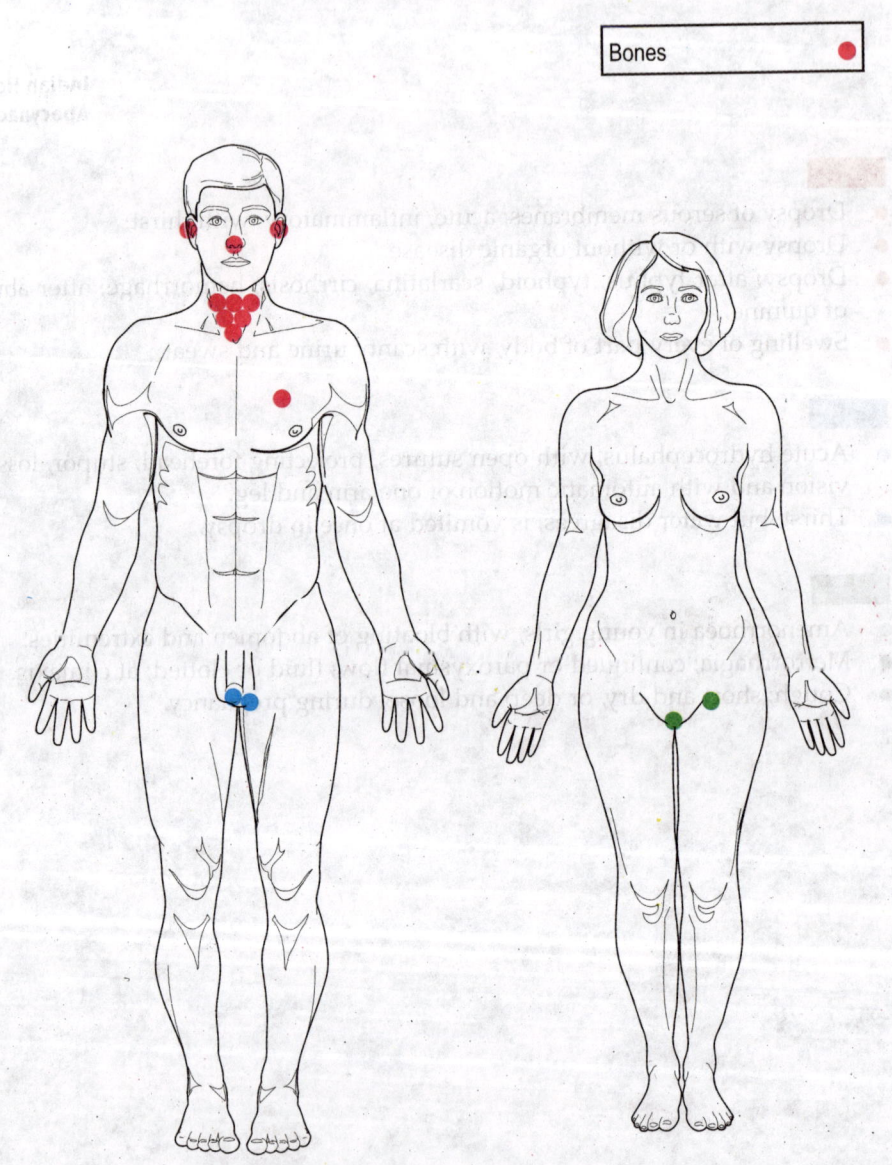

Bones ●

40 A

ARGENTUM METALLICUM

Pure Silver
Ag

- Hoarseness and aphonia; of professional singers, public speakers < using voice.
- Alteration in timber of voice with singers and public speakers.
- When reading aloud has to hem and hawk.
- Laughing excites cough and produces profuse mucus in larynx.
- Easy expectoration of gray, gelatinous or starchy mucus.
- Raw spot over bifurcation of the trachea.
- Great weakness of the chest; worse left side.
- Affects the cartilages, tarsi, ears, nose, Eustachian; bones, condyles, ligaments, the structures entering into joints.

- Seminal emissions: after onanism; almost every night; without erection; with atrophy of penis.
- Crushed pain in the testicles.

- Prolapsus uteri: with pain in left ovary and back, extending forward and downward; climacteric hemorrhage.

SURFACE MARKING OF KEYNOTES

ARGENTUM NITRICUM

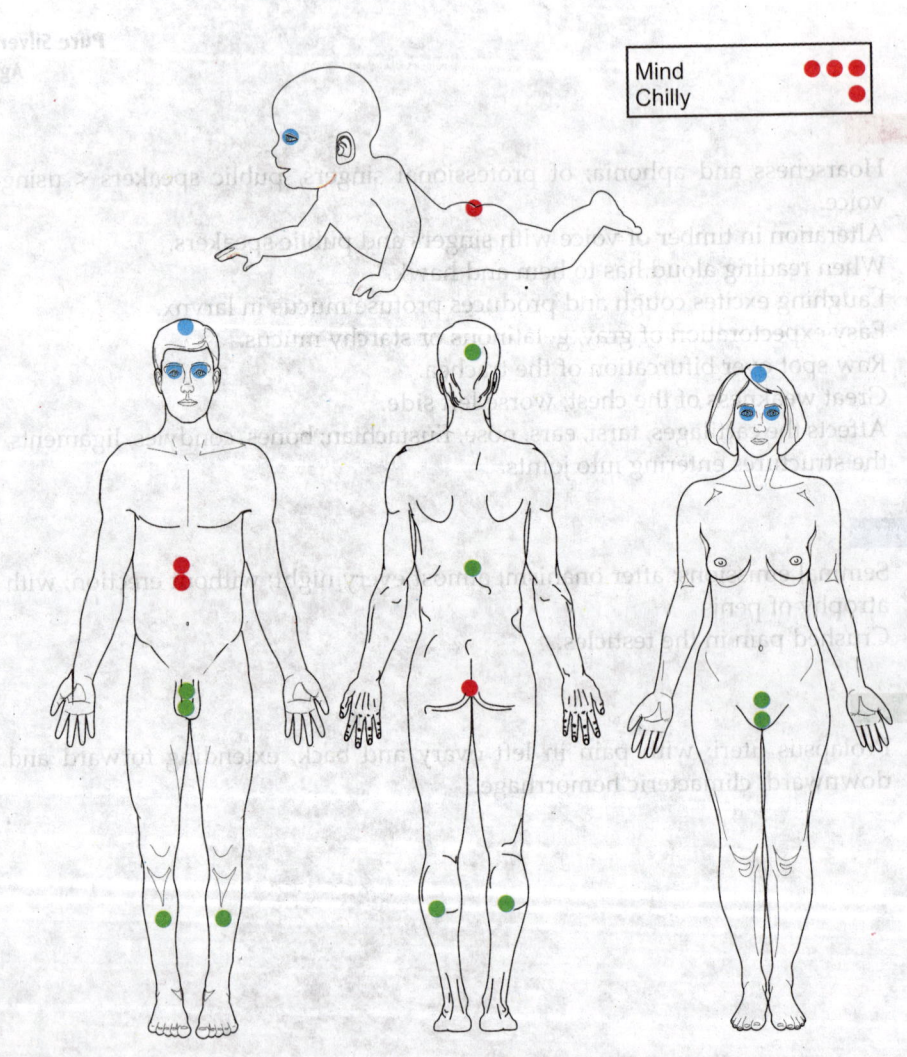

42 A

ARGENTUM NITRICUM

The Silver Nitrate
AgNO$_3$

- Acute or chronic diseases from unusual or long-continued mental exertion.
- Apprehension when ready for church or opera, diarrhea sets in.
- Time passes slowly; impulsive, wants to do things in a hurry.
- Chilly when uncovered, yet feels smothered if wrapped up; craves fresh air.
- Belching accompanies most gastric ailments.
- Flatulent dyspepsia; stomach; as if it would burst with wind.
- Diarrhea; green mucus, like chopped spinach in flakes; turning green after remaining on diaper; after drinking; after eating candy or sugar.

- Headache with sense of expansion; from dancing; < from any exhaustive mental labor; > by pressure or tight bandaging.
- Acute granular conjunctivitis; scarlet-red, like raw beef; discharge profuse, muco-purulent.
- Ophthalmia neonatorum; profuse, purulent discharge.
- Cornea opaque, ulcerated.
- Lids sore, thick, swollen; agglutinated in morning.
- Eye strain from sewing, < in warm room, > in open air.
- Diseases due to defective accommodation.

- Disseminated sclerosis of brain and cord.
- Great weakness of lower extremities; with trembling.
- Walks and stands unsteadily.
- Impotence; erection fails when coition is attempted.
- Coition: painful in both sexes; followed by bleeding from vagina.
- Metrorrhagia: in young widows and childless women; with nervous erethism at change of life.

SURFACE MARKING OF KEYNOTES

ARNICA MONTANA

Injuries ●●●●
Pain
Mind
Paralysis
Rheumatism
Fever
Skin

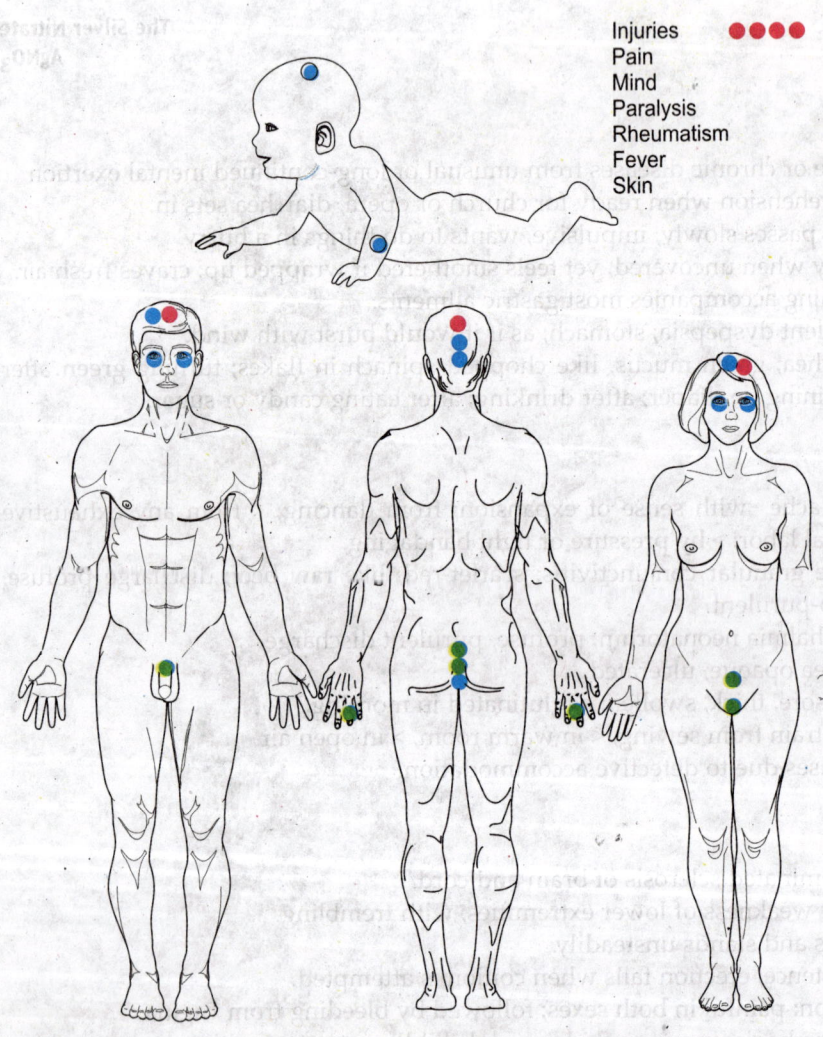

44 A

ARNICA MONTANA

Leopard's Bane
Compositae

- Sore, lame, bruised feeling all through the body, as if beaten.
- Mechanical injuries, especially with stupor from concussion.
- Concussions and contusions, results of shock or injury; without laceration of soft parts; prevents suppuration and septic conditions and promotes absorption.
- After injuries with blunt instruments.
- Compound fractures and their profuse suppuration.
- Everything on which he lies seems too hard.
- Heat of upper part of body; coldness of lower.

- Conjunctival or retinal haemorrhage, with extravasations, from injuries or cough.
- Hydrocephalus: with deathly coldness in forearm of children.
- Meningitis after mechanical or traumatic injuries; from falls, concussion of brain etc.
- Apoplexy: loss of consciousness, involuntary, evacuation from bowels and bladder.
- Paralysis, left sided.

- Gout and rheumatism, with great fear of being touched or struck by persons coming near him.
- Soreness of parts after labor; prevents post-partum haemorrhage and puerperal complications.
- Retention or incontinence of urine after labor.
- Dysentery; with ischuria, fruitless urging; long interval between the stools..
- Constipation: rectum loaded, faeces will not come away; ribbon-like stools from enlarged prostate or retroverted uterus.
- Intermittent, typhoid, septic, traumatic fevers.
- Very sore acne or crops of small boils.

SURFACE MARKING OF KEYNOTES

ARSENICUM ALBUM

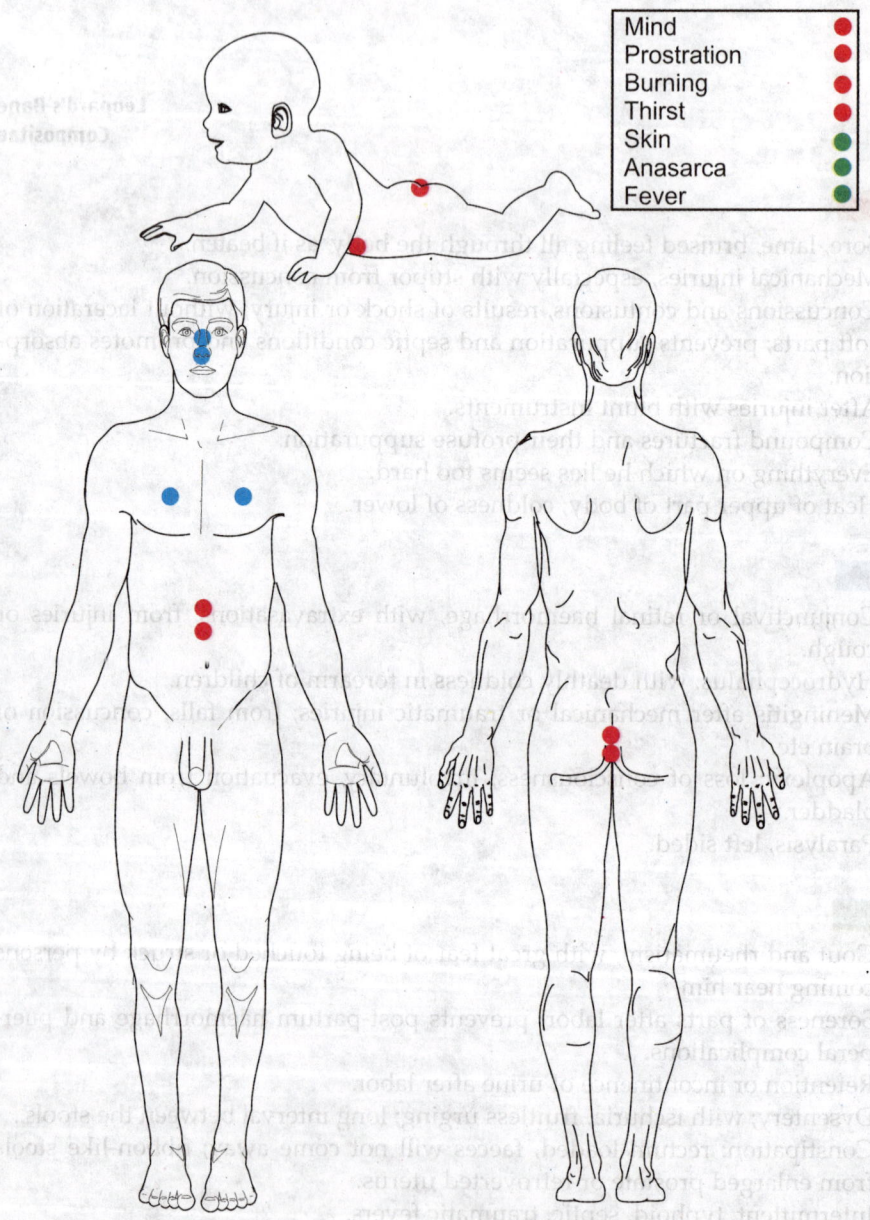

Mind	🔴
Prostration	🔴
Burning	🔴
Thirst	🔴
Skin	🟢
Anasarca	🟢
Fever	🟢

46 A

ARSENICUM ALBUM

White Oxide of Arsenic
As_2O_3

- Mentally restless, but physically too weak to move; cannot rest in any place.
- Great prostration, with rapid sinking of the vital forces; fainting.
- Burning pains; the affected parts burn like fire, > by heat, hot drinks, hot applications.
- Symptoms generally worse from 1-2 p.m., 12-2 a.m.
- Great thirst for cold water; drinks often, but little at a time; eats seldom, but much.
- Gastric derangements; after cold fruits; ice-cream; ice water; sour beer; bad sausage; alcoholic drinks; strong cheese.
- Diarrhea, after eating or drinking; stool scanty; dark-colored, offensive, followed by great prostration.
- Dysentery, cholera, in children.

- Bad effects from decayed food or animal matter, whether by inoculation, olfaction or ingestion.
- Cannot bear the sight or smell of food.
- Thin, watery, excoriating discharge from nose with sneezing.
- Breathing: asthmatic; must sit or bend forward; springs out of bed at night, especially after 12 O'clock; unable to lie down for fear of suffocation.

- Destructive process - Carbuncles, gangrene, cancer; malignancy.
- Anasarca; skin pale, puffy, baggy, waxy, earth-colored.
- Intermittent fever, yellow fever, typhoid fever.

SURFACE MARKING OF KEYNOTES

ARSENICUM IODATUM

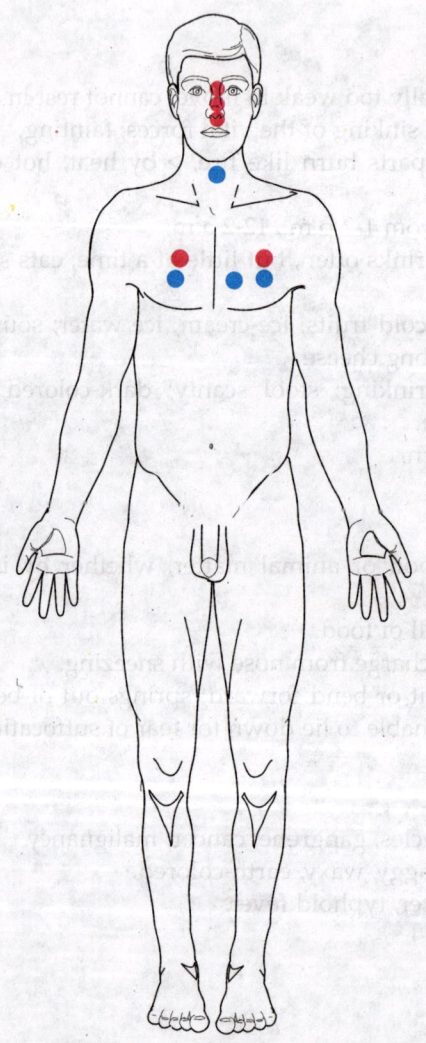

ARSENICUM IODATUM

Iodide of Arsenic
AsI$_3$

- Thin, watery, irritating, excoriating discharge from anterior and posterior nares; sneezing.
- Chronic nasal catarrh; swollen nose; profuse, thick yellow discharge; ulcers; membrane sore and excoriated.
- Hay fever, Influenza.
- Early stage of tuberculosis, with afternoon rise of temperature.
- Recurrent fever and drenching night-sweats.

- Hoarseness. Aphonia.
- Short of breath; air hunger.
- Pneumonia that fails to clear up.
- Senile heart, myocarditis and fatty degeneration.

- Psoriasis, Icthyosis.
- Marked exfoliation of skin in large scales leaving a exudating surface beneath.
- Enlarged scrofulous glands.

SURFACE MARKING OF KEYNOTES

ARUM TRIPHYLLUM

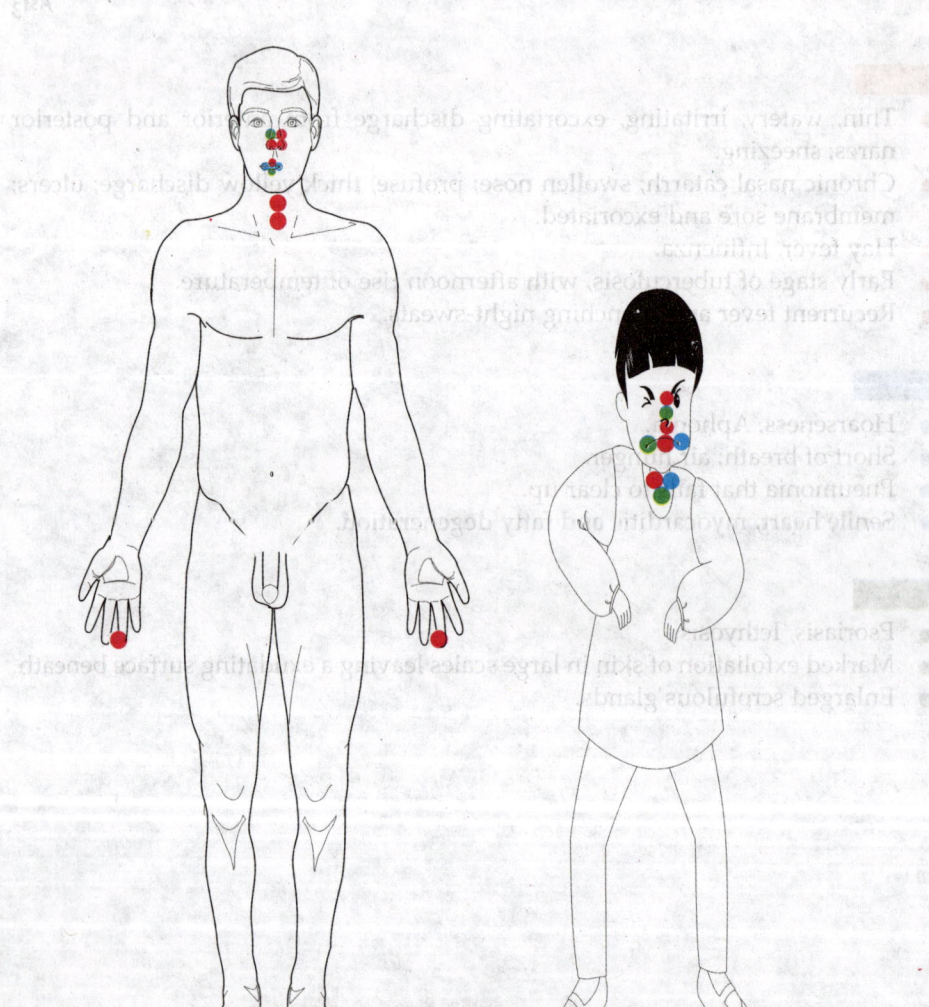

ARUM TRIPHYLLUM

Indian Turnip
Araceae

- Patients pick and bore into the raw bleeding surfaces though very painful; scream with pain but keep up the boring.
- Persistantly boring into nose; or pricking at lips, fingers, at one spot until it is sore or bleeds, esp. children.
- Coryza: acrid, fluent, ichorous, excoriating; nostrils raw.
- Nose feels stopped up inspite of the watery discharge; sneezing < at night.
- Aphonia: complete, after exposure to northwest winds; from singing.
- Clergyman's sore throat; voice hoarse, uncertain, uncontrollable, changing continually; worse from talking, speaking or singing; orators, singers, actors.

- Corners of mouth sore, cracked, bleeding.
- Saliva profuse, acrid, corrodes the mucous membrane; tongue and buccal cavity raw and bleeding.
- Children refuse food and drink on account of soreness of mouth and throat; are sleepless.

- The sore mouth and nose are guiding in malignant scarlatina and diphtheria.
- Desquamation in large flakes; a second or third time, in scarlatina.

SURFACE MARKING OF KEYNOTES

AURUM METALLICUM

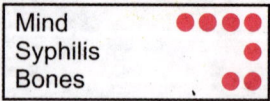

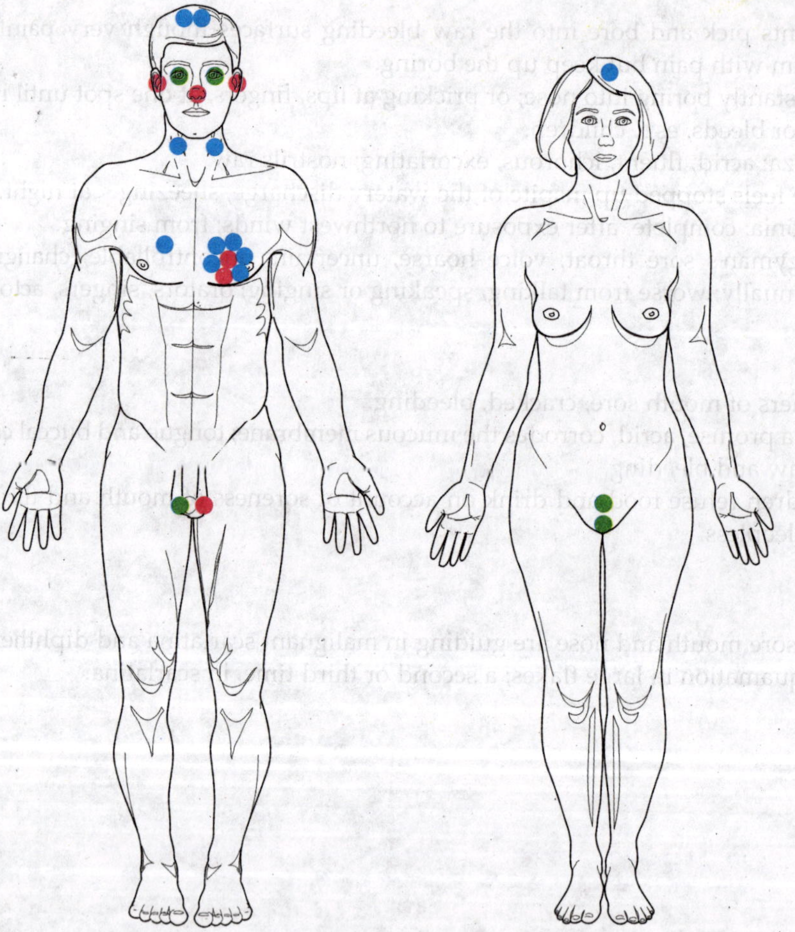

52 A

AURUM METALLICUM

Gold
Au

- It is adapted to nervous, hysterical women; girls at puberty; pining boys with undeveloped testes; old people with heart disease; to persons who are low-spirited, lifeless, weak memory; yet sensitive to pain; which drives them to despair.
- Constantly dwelling on suicide.
- Profound melancholy; with nearly all complaints.
- Syphilitic and mercurial affections of the bones.
- Caries of bones especially of nose, palatine and mastoid.
- Hopeless with heart disease; hopeful with lung disease.

- Headache; from least mental exertion; with constipation.
- Baldness from syphilis.
- Sensation as if the heart stopped beating, immediately followed by hard rebound.
- Violent palpitation; anxiety, with congestion of blood to head and chest after exertion.
- Visible beating of carotid and temporal arteries.
- High blood pressure.
- Fatty degeneration of heart.

- Hemiopia; sees only the lower half.
- Chronic induration of testicles.
- Prolapsed and indurated uterus; from over - reaching or straining; from hypertrophy.
- Syphilitic sterility.

BAPTISIA TINCTORIA

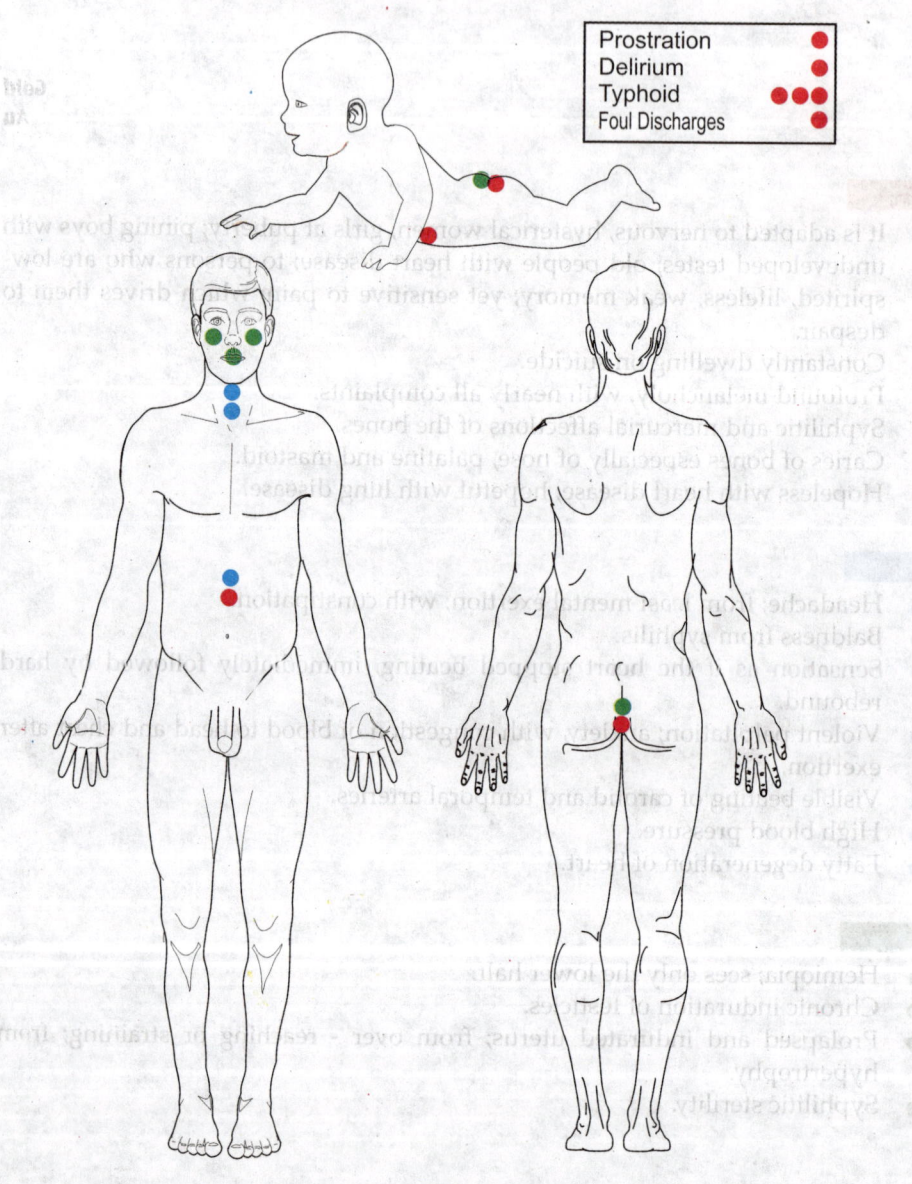

BAPTISIA TINCTORIA

Wild Indigo
Leguminosae

- Great prostration, with disposition to decomposition of fluids; ulceration of mucous membranes.
- All exhalations and discharges fetid, especially in typhoid or other acute disease; breath, stool, urine, perspiration, ulcer.
- Stupor: falls asleep while being spoken to or in the midst of his answer.
- Decubitus in typhoid.
- In whatever position the patient lies, the parts rested upon feel sore and bruised.

- Can swallow liquids only; least solid food gags.
- Painless sore throat; tonsils, soft palate and parotids dark red, swollen; putrid, offensive discharge.

- Tongue: at first coated white with red papillae; dry and yellow-brown in centre; later dry, cracked, ulcerated.
- Dysentery of old people; painless, with fever; offensive.
- Diarrhea of children; painless; sudden, horribly foul.
- Face flushed, dusky, dark colored, with a stupid, be-sotted drunken expression.

SURFACE MARKING OF KEYNOTES

BARYTA CARBONICA

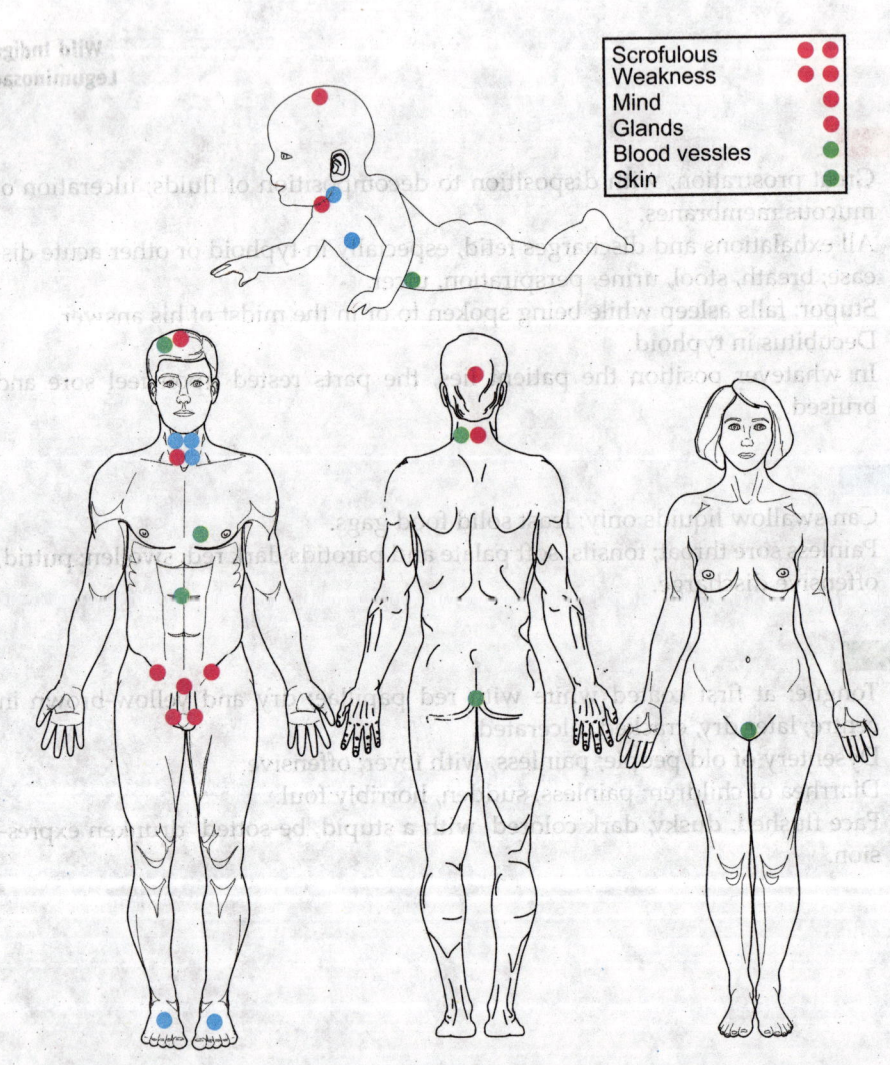

Scrofulous	● ●
Weakness	● ●
Mind	●
Glands	●
Blood vessels	●
Skin	●

BARYTA CARBONICA

Barium Carbonate
BaCo$_3$

- Pre-eminently a remedy for children and the elderly.
- Scrofulous, dwarfish children who do not grow.
- Children both physically and mentally weak.
- Memory deficient; threatened idiocy.
- Old, cachectic people; scrofulous, especially when fat; mental and physical weakness; who are childish.
- Diseases of old men; hypertrophy or induration of prostate and testes; gouty complaints; headache; apoplectic tendency.
- Swelling and indurations, or incipient suppuration of glands, especially tonsils, cervical and inguinal.

- Persons subject to quinsy, take cold easily, even the least cold precipitates an attack of tonsillitis, prone to suppuration.
- Inability to swallow anything but liquids.
- Chronic cough in psoric children.
- Cold, offensive foot sweat.
- Throat affections after checked foot sweat.

- Vascular softening, dilatation and degenerative changes—aneurism, ruptures, apoplexy, arteriosclerosis.
- High blood pressure.
- Lipoma. Fatty tumors upon the neck.
- Cysts. Burning sarcoma.
- Menses scanty, last only one day.
- Habitual colic of children.
- Dyspepsia of young masturbators.
- Piles protrude, while urinating.

SURFACE MARKING OF KEYNOTES

BELLADONNA

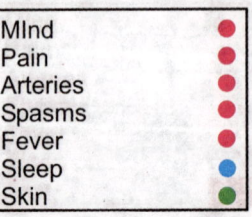

- Mind
- Pain
- Arteries
- Spasms
- Fever
- Sleep
- Skin

58 B

BELLADONNA

Deadly Nightshade
Solanaceae

- Women and children with light hair and blue eyes, fine complexion, delicate skin; sensitive, nervous, threatened with convulsions.
- Violent delirium; disposition to bite, spit, strike and tear things.
- Great liability to take cold.
- Severe neuralgic pain, that comes and goes suddenly; in short attacks.
- Congestion, throbbing, and dilatation of arteries.
- Burning heat, bright redness and dryness are very marked.
- Spasms, shocks; jerks and twitchings.
- Convulsions during teething, with fever.
- Discharges are hot and scanty.

- Rush of blood to head and face.
- Headache; hammering, congestive, with red face, throbbing of brain and carotids; < motion, > pressure.
- Boring the head into the pillow.
- Eyes; wild, staring, pupils dilated; red conjunctiva; photophobia.
- High fever; hot head, with cold limbs.
- Internal coldness, with external pungent, burning, steaming heat.
- Sleepy but cannot sleep.

- Skin: of a uniform, smooth, shining scarlet redness.
- Acts as a prophylactic in scarlet fever.
- Tonsils; enlarged, inflamed < cold wind.
- Abdomen tender, distended < by least jar, even of the bed.
- Prolapsus uteri; > standing and sitting erect, < lying down, mornings.
- Hematuria without pathological conditions.
- Exophthalmic goiter, with extreme thyroid toxaemia.

SURFACE MARKING OF KEYNOTES

BERBERIS VULGARIS

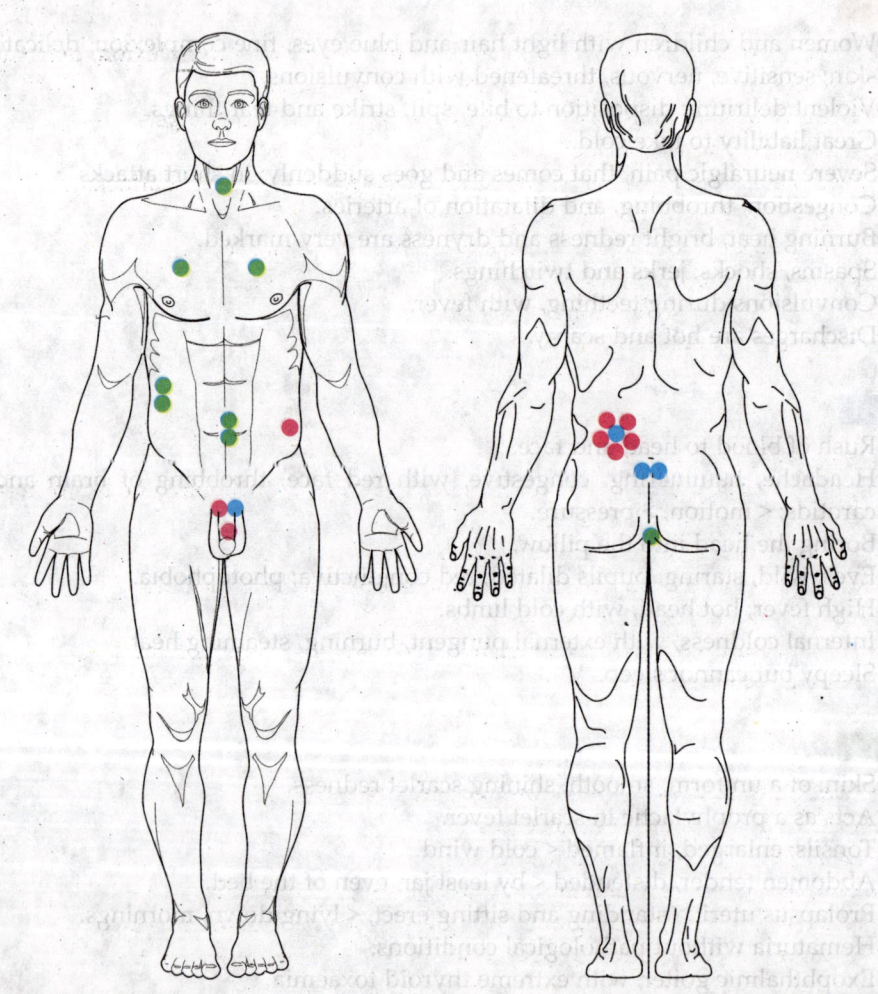

60 B

BERBERIS VULGARIS

Barberry
Berberidaceae

- The renal or vesical symptoms predominate.
- Renal colic, < left side.
- Stitching, cutting pain from left kidney following course of ureter into bladder and urethra.
- Burning and soreness in region of kidneys.
- Bubbling sensation in kidneys.

- Rheumatic and gouty complaints, with diseases of the urinary organs.
- Pains rapidly change their locality and character.
- Pain in small of back; very sensitive to touch in renal region; < when sitting and lying, from jar, from fatigue.
- Numbness, stiffness, lameness with painful pressure in renal and lumbar regions.
- Urine: greenish, blood red, with thick, turbid, slimy mucus, transparent, reddish or jelly-like sediment.

- Colic from gall-stones.
- Bilious colic, followed by jaundice; clay colored stools.
- Promotes the flow of bile.
- Fistula in ano, with bilious symptoms and itching of the parts.
- Short cough and chest complaints, especially after operations for fistulae.

SURFACE MARKING OF KEYNOTES

BISMUTHUM

Mind ● ●

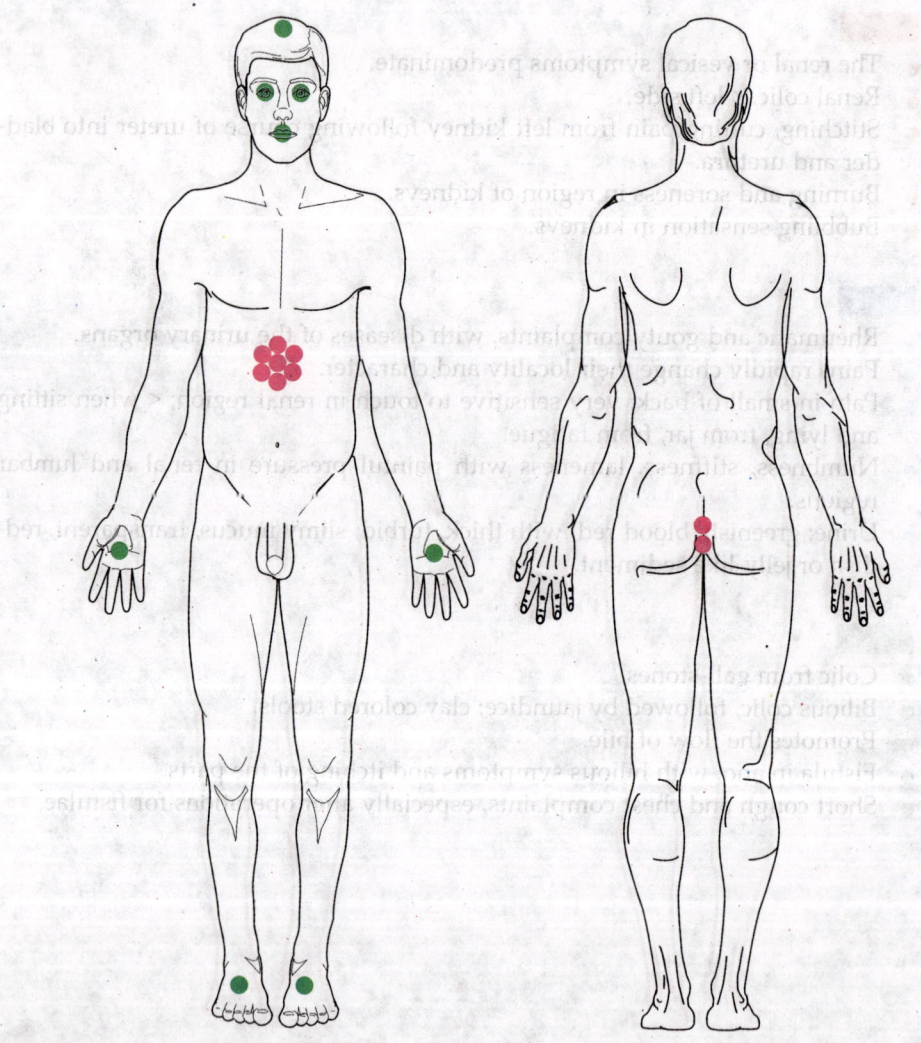

62 B

BISMUTHUM

Hydrated Oxide of Bismuth
Bi$_2$ O$_3$ OH$_2$

- Vomiting: of water as soon as it reaches the stomach, food retained longer.
- Vomits all fluids as soon as taken.
- Vomiting of enormous quantities, as intervals of several days when food has filled the stomach.
- Vomiting with convulsive gagging and inexpressible pain, after laparotomy or abdominal operations.
- Cancer of stomach, vomiting of brownish water.
- Food presses like a load in one spot.
- Cholera morbis and summer complaint, when vomiting predominates.
- Stools; papescent, watery, offensive, very prostrating, painless, with thirst, frequent vomiting and micturition.

- Solitude is unbearable: desires company, child holds on to its mother's hand for company.
- Anguish; he sits, then walks, then lies, never long in one place.

- Face, deathly pale, blue rings around the eyes.
- Headache returning every winter; alternating with, or attended by gastralgia.
- Toothache > by holding cold water in mouth < when it becomes warm.
- Dry palms and soles.

SURFACE MARKING OF KEYNOTES

BORAX

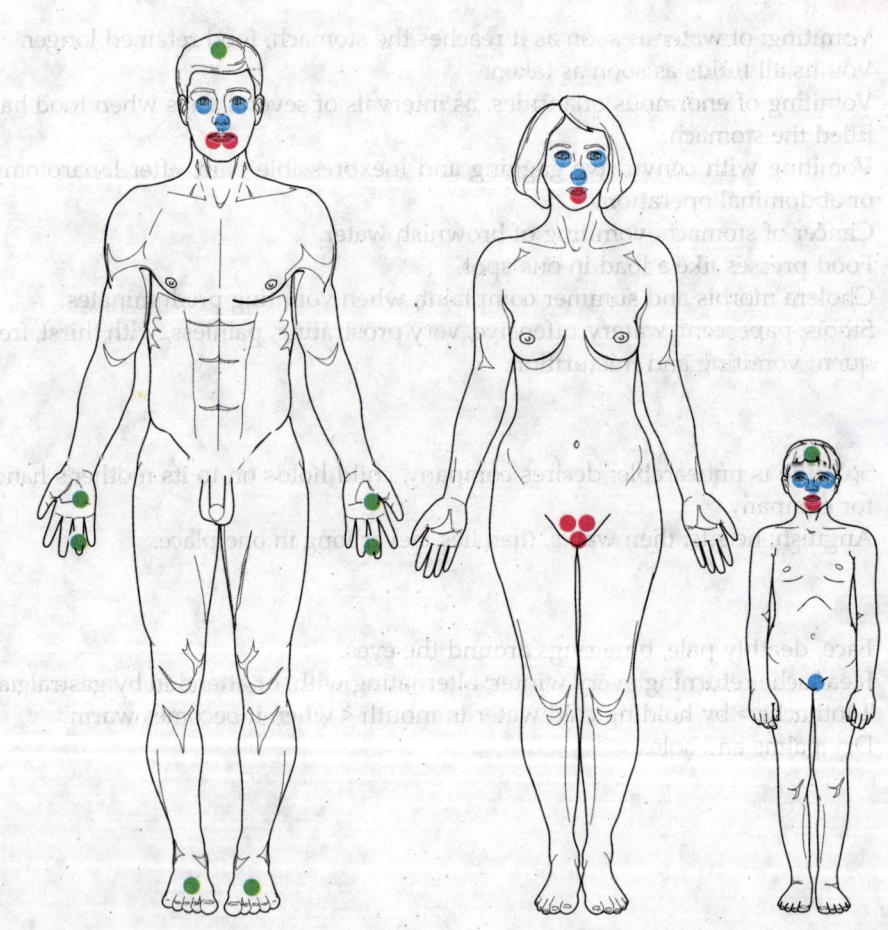

64 B

BORAX

Biborate of Soda
$Na_2B_4O_7 \cdot 10H_2O$

- Dread of downward motion in nearly all complaints; when rocking, dancing, swinging; going down stairs, or rapidly down hill.
- Excessively nervous, easily frightened by the slightest noise or an unusual sharp sound.
- Aphthous sore mouth; is worse from touch; eating salty or sour food; of old people, often from plate of teeth.
- Aphthae; in the mouth, on the tongue, inside of the cheek; easily bleeding when eating or touched; with hot mouth, dryness and thirst.
- Aphthae prevents child from nursing.
- Leucorrhoea; profuse, albuminous, starchy, with sensation as if warm water were flowing down; for two weeks between the menstruation.
- Membranous dysmenorrhoea.
- Sterility, favours easy conception.

- Eyelids; loaded with dry, gummy exudation; agglutinated in morning.
- Eyelashes; turn inward and inflame the eye, especially at outer canthus; tendency to "wild hairs." Entropion.
- Red noses of young women.
- Nostrils crusty, inflamed; tip of nose shining red.
- Stoppage of nostrils alternately; with lachrymation.
- Child has frequent urination and screams before urine passes.

- Hair entangled at tips, stick together cannot be separated or combed smooth.
- Skin unhealthy, slight injuries suppurate.
- Trade eruptions, on fingers and hands, itching and stinging eczema.
- Ulceration on feet from rubbing of shoe.

SURFACE MARKING OF KEYNOTES

BOVISTA

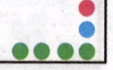

Haemorrhage	●
Mind	●
Skin	●●●●

66 B

BOVISTA

Puffball
Fungi

- Discharge from nose and all mucous membranes very tough, stringy, tenacious.
- Hemorrhage: after extraction of teeth; from wounds; epistaxis.
- Menses: flow only at night; not in the daytime; less while moving; occasional show every few day between periods, early, every two weeks, dark and clotted; with painful bearing down.
- Diarrhea before or during menses.

- Stammering children.
- Awkwardness, inclined to drop things from hands; objects fall from powerless hands.
- Great weakness of joints and weariness of hands and feet.
- Visible palpitation of heart; of old maids.

- A general puffiness and bloated condition of body surface, which produces easy indentations or deep impression usually on finger, from using blunt instruments like scissors, knife, etc.
- Intolerable itching at tip of coccyx, must scratch till parts become raw and sore.
- Itching eruptions; oozing; forming thick crusts, scabs, with pus beneath.
- Urticaria covering whole body, with diarrhea or metrorrhagia.

SURFACE MARKING OF KEYNOTES

BROMIUM

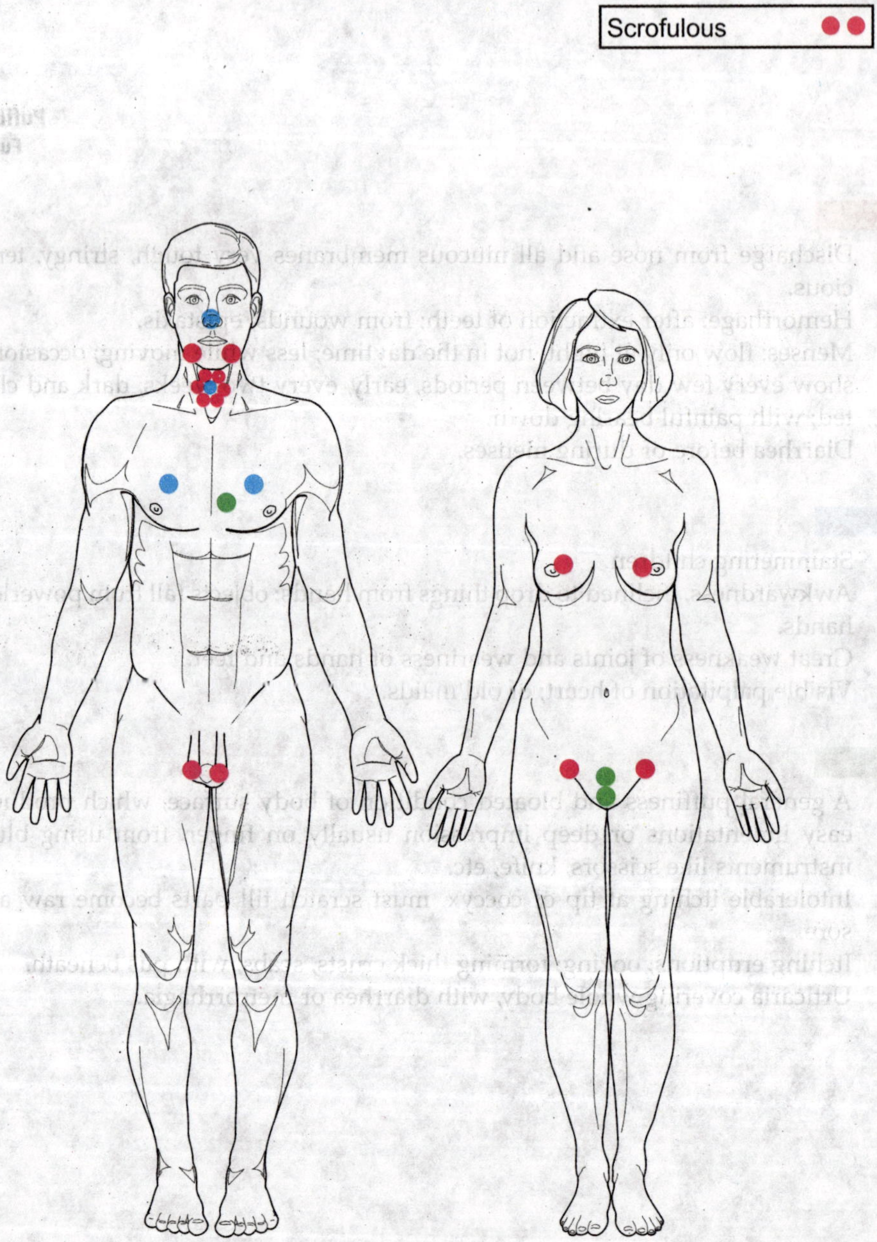

Scrofulous

68 B

BROMIUM

Bromine
Br

- Persons with light-blue eyes, flaxen hair, light eyebrows, fair, delicate skin; blonde, red-cheeked, scrofulous girls.
- Patient is week and easily overheated; then sweaty and sensitive to drafts.
- Stony, hard, scrofulous or tuberculous swelling of glands, especially on lower jaw and throat-thyroid, submaxillary, parotid, testes, ovaries and mammary glands.
- Diphtheria: where the membrane forms in pharynx; beginning in bronchi, trachea or larynx, and extending upwards; chest pains running upwards.
- Membranous and diphtheritic croup; much rattling of mucus during cough, but no choking.
- Croupy symptoms with hoarseness during whooping cough; gasping for breath.
- Cold sensation in larynx on inspiration; > after shaving.

- Sailors suffer from asthma. "on shore".
- Dyspnoea: cannot inspire deep enough; as if breathing through a sponge or the air passages were full of smoke.
- Danger of suffocation from mucus in larynx.
- Fan-like motion of alae nasi.

- Hypertrophy of heart from: gymnastics in growing boys, with palpitation.
- Physometra; loud emission of flatus from the vagina.
- Membranous dysmenorrhoea.

SURFACE MARKING OF KEYNOTES

BRYONIA ALBA

Mind	●
Pain	●
Modalities	●
Thirst	●
Rheumatism	●
Fever	●

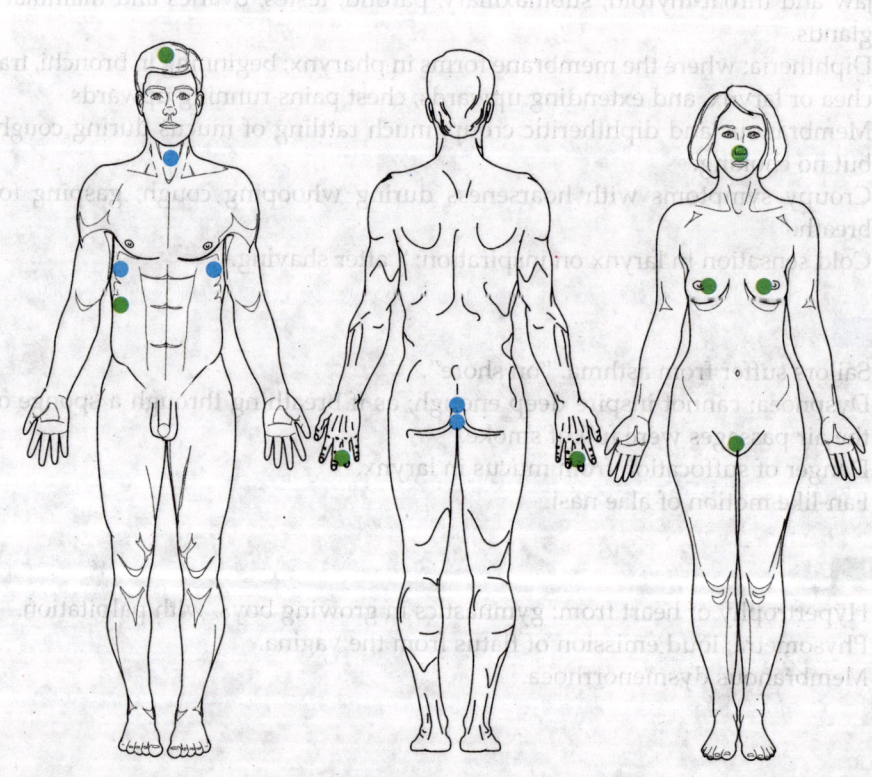

70 B

BRYONIA ALBA

White Bryony, Wild Hop
Cucurbitaceae

- Ailments from chagrin, mortification, anger; after anger chilly, but with head hot and face red.
- Complaints: when warm weather sets in, after cold days; after taking cold or getting hot in summer; from exposure to draft, cold wind; suppressed discharges, or eruption.
- Pains: stitching, tearing, worse at night; < by motion, inspiration, coughing; > by absolute rest, and lying or painful side.
- Excessive dryness of mucous membranes of entire body.
- One of the chief characteristics of *Bryonia* is aggravation from any motion, and corresponding relief from absolute rest, either mental or physical.
- Great thirst for large quantities at long intervals.

- Cough: dry, hard, racking, spasmodic, with gagging and vomiting with stitches inside of chest; with scanty expectoration < after eating, drinking, entering a warm room, a deep inspiration.
- Constipation: inactive, no inclination; stool large, hard, dark, dry as if burnt; on going to sea.
- Diarrhea: during a spell of hot weather; < in morning, on moving, even a hand or foot.

- Gouty or rheumatic diathesis.
- Headache: when stooping.
- Mammae heavy, of a stony hardness; pale but hard; hot and painful; must support the breast.
- Vicarious menstruation: nosebleed when menses should appear.
- Typhoid, bilious, rheumatic and remittent types of fevers.

SURFACE MARKING OF KEYNOTES

CACTUS GRANDIFLORUS

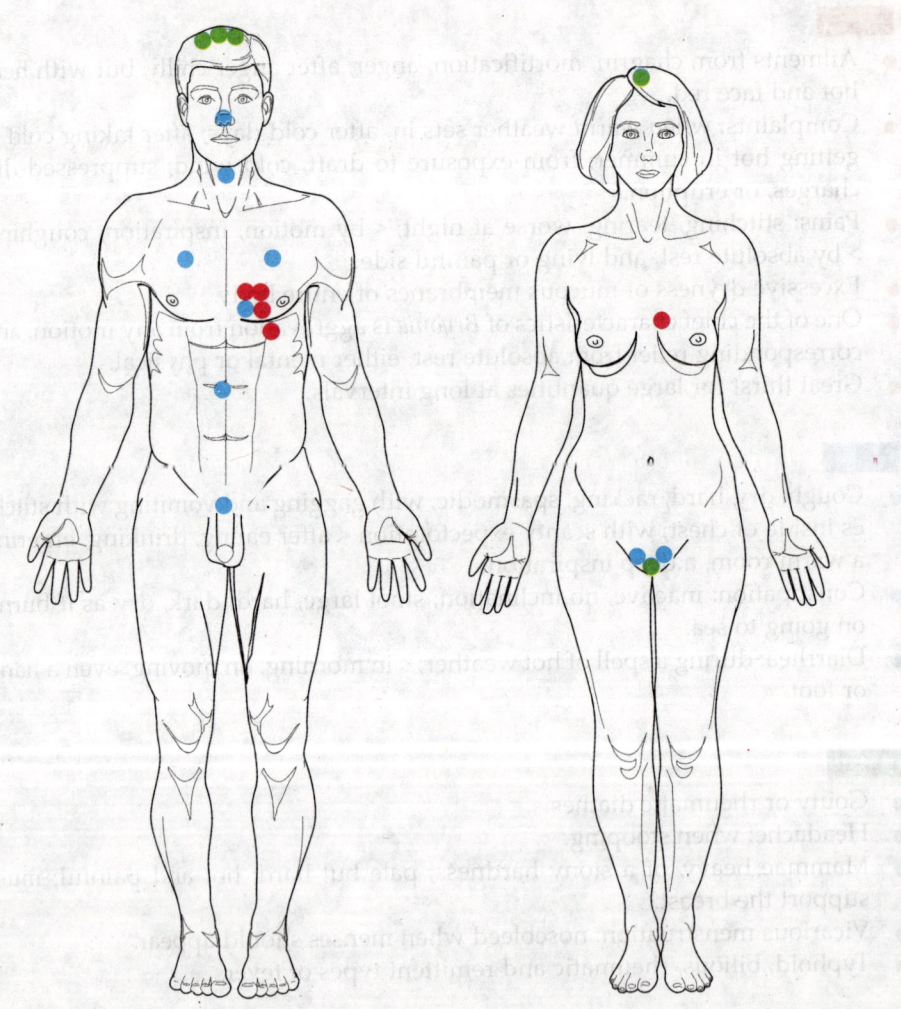

72 C

CACTUS GRANDIFLORUS

Night-blooming Cereus
Cactaceae

- Whole body feels as if caged, each wire being twisted tighter and tighter.
- Oppression of chest, as from a great weight; as if an iron band prevented normal motion.
- Sensation of a cord tightly tied around lower part of chest, marking attachment of diaphragm.
- Heart feels as if clasped and unclasped rapidly by an iron hand; as if bound; darting, springing like chain lightning, and ending with a sharp, vise-like grip, only to be again renewed.
- Palpitation: day and night; worse when walking and lying on left side; at approach of menses.

- Fear of death; believes the disease incurable.
- Hemorrhage: from nose, lungs, stomach, rectum, bladder.
- It affects the circular muscles, there by producing constrictions; of the heart, throat, chest, bladder, rectum, uterus, vagina, neck; often caused or brought on by the slightest contact.

- Sanguineous apoplexy.
- Headache, pressing like a heavy weight on vertex; climacteric.
- Headache and neuralgia; congestive, periodic, right-sided; severe, throbbing, pulsating pain.
- Menstrual flow ceases when lying down.
- Fever paroxysm at 11 a.m. and 11 p.m.

SURFACE MARKING OF KEYNOTES

CALCAREA ARSENICA

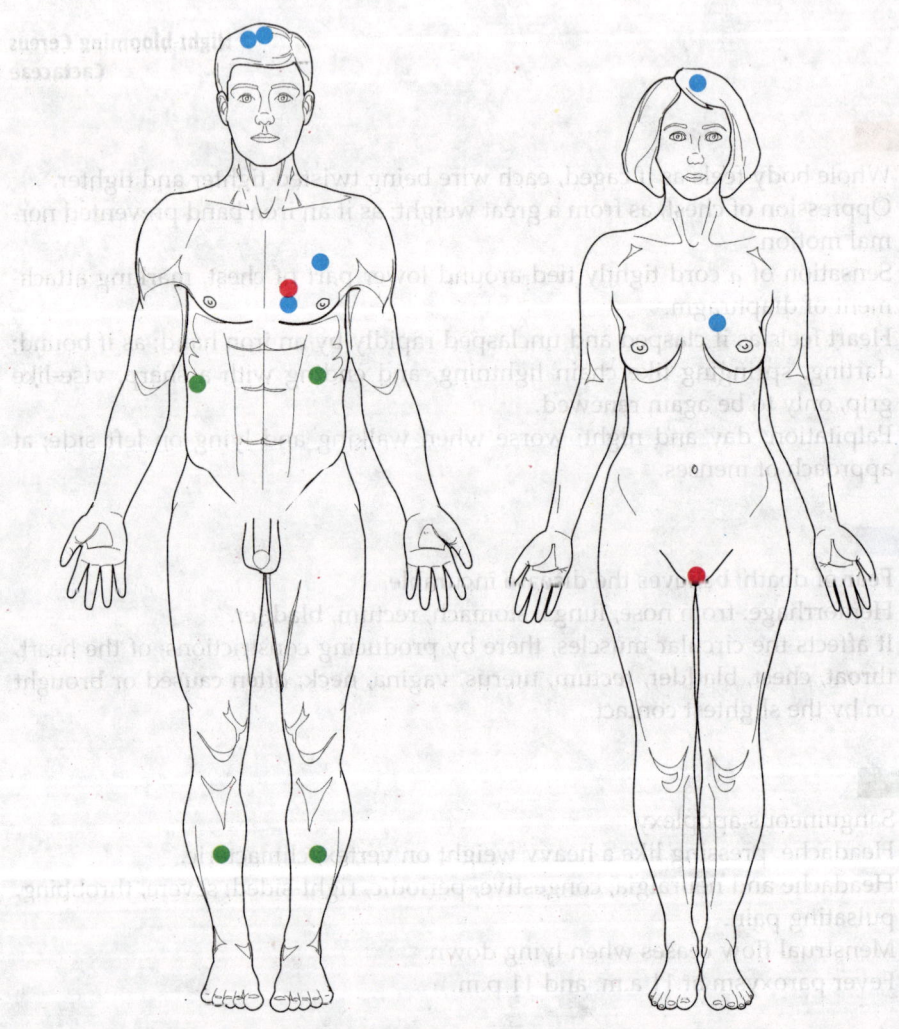

CALCAREA ARSENICA

Arsenite of Lime
$Ca_3(AsO_3)_2$

- Complaints of fleshy women when approaching the menopause.
- The slightest emotion causes palpitation of heart.

- Rush of blood to head and left chest.
- Epilepsies, from valvular diseases of the heart.
- Palpitation and heart pains before epileptic attack.
- Relieves burning pain in cancer.

- Complaints of drunkards, after abstaining; craving for alcohol.
- Enlarged liver and spleen in chronic malaria; in children.
- Removes inflammatory products in veins of lower limbs.

SURFACE MARKING OF KEYNOTES

CALCAREA CARBONICA

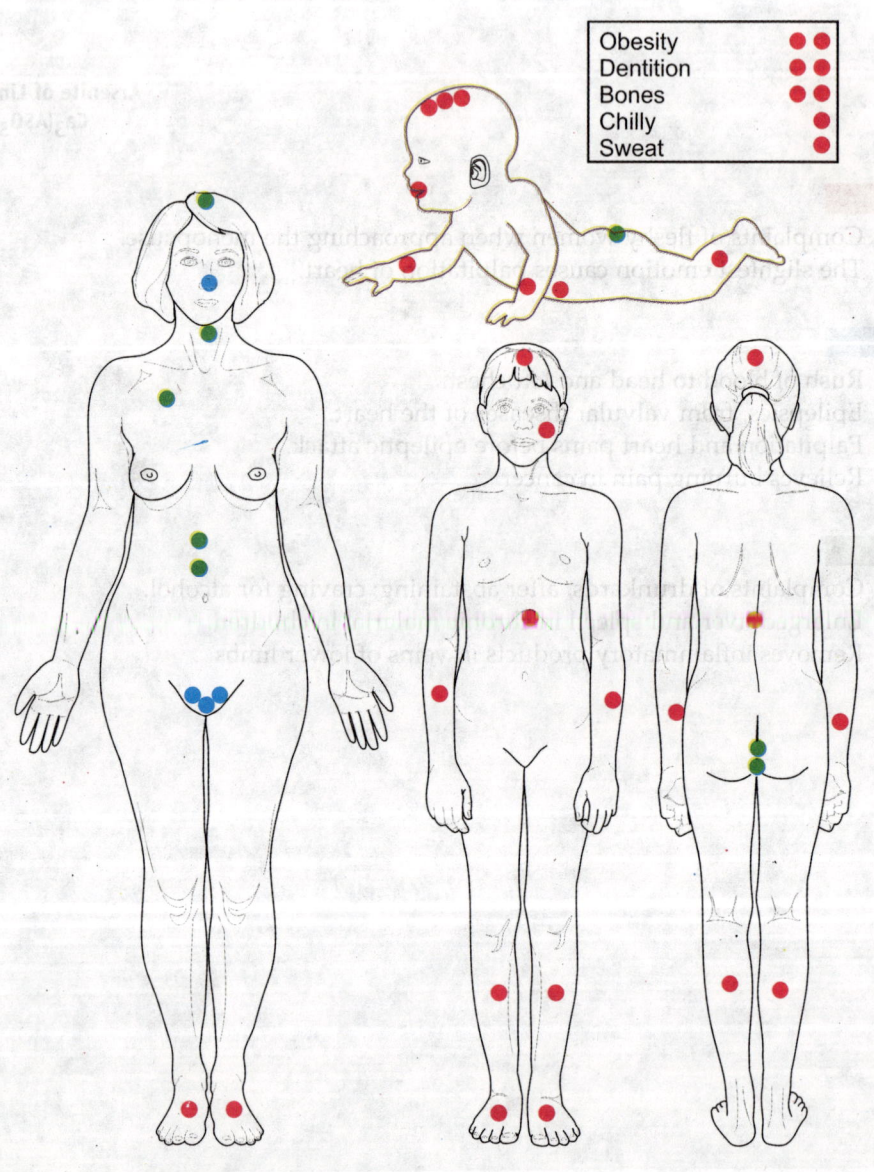

76 C

CALCAREA CARBONICA

Middle Layer of Oyster Shell
Calcium Carbonate

- Calcarea patient can be described as fat, flabby, fair, forty, perspiring, cold and damp.
- Disposed to grow fat, corpulent, unwieldy.
- Children with red face, flabby muscles, when sweat easily.
- Difficult and delayed dentition with characteristic head sweats.
- Large heads and abdomens; fontanelles and sutures open; bones soft, develop very slowly.
- Curvature of bones, especially spine and long bones; extremities crooked, deformed; bones irregularly developed.
- Head sweats profusely while sleeping, wetting pillow far around.
- Diseases: arising from defective assimilation; imperfect ossification; difficulty in learning to walk or stand.
- Coldness: general; of single parts; great liability to take cold.
- Great longing for eggs; craves indigestible things; aversion to meat.
- Sweat: of single parts; offensive foot sweat.
- Feet habitually cold and damp, as if they had on cold damp stockings.

- Girls who are fleshy, plethoric, and grow too rapidly.
- Menstruation too early, too profuse, too long lasting; with subsequent amenorrhoea and chlorosis with menses scanty or suppressed.
- The least mental excitement causes profuse return of menstrual flow or brings on dysmenorrhoea.
- Polypi; nasal, uterine etc.

- Lung diseases of tall, slender, rapidly growing youth; upper third of right lung.
- Acidity of digestive tract; sour eructation, sour vomiting, sour stool.
- Pit of stomach swollen like an inverted saucer, and painful to pressure.
- Stool has to be removed mechanically.
- Feels better in every way when constipated.
- Sour odor of the whole body.
- Pituitary and thyroid dysfunction.
- Osteomylitis. Epilepsy. Uraemia. Urticaria.

SURFACE MARKING OF KEYNOTES

CALCAREA FLUORICA

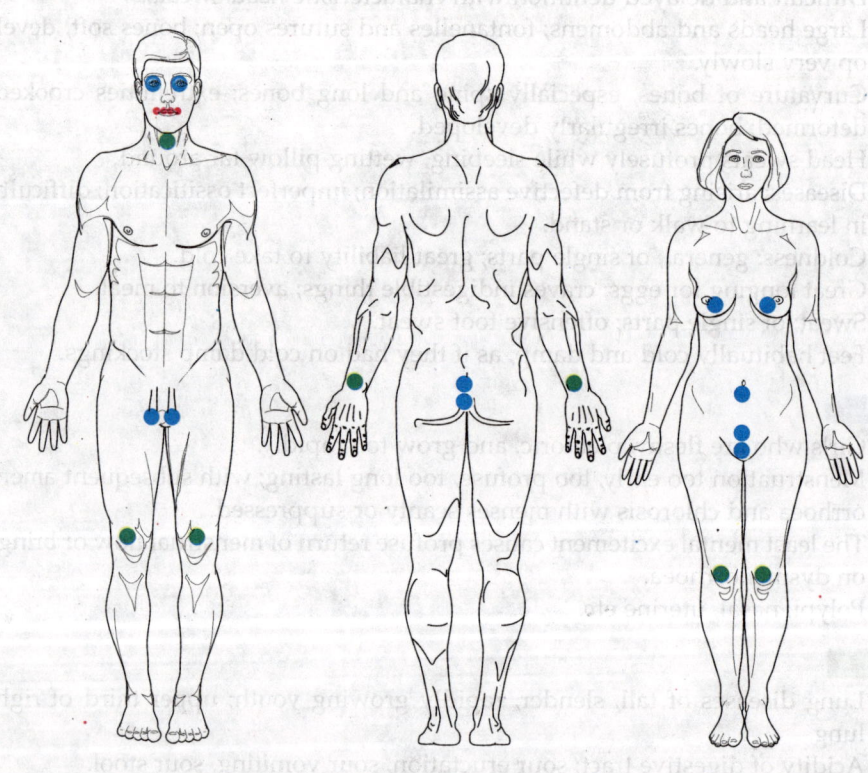

Glands
Veins
Skin

CALCAREA FLUORICA

Fluoride of Lime
CaF$_2$

- Glands enlarge and become stony hard.
- Veins; dilated; varicose or enlarged; inflamed.
- Swelling and indurations around tendons and joints.
- Gumboil, with hard swelling of the jaw. Pyorrhea.
- Deficient enamel of teeth.
- Teeth become loose in their sockets.
- Toothache, if any food touches the tooth.

- Cataract
- Bleeding piles; with pain in sacrum.
- Constipation. Flatulency. Fissures. Fistula.
- Hydrocele. Indurated testes.
- Hard knots in mammae.
- Favors easy confinement.
- Hanging belly or pendulous abdomen.
- Uterine displacement.

- Laryngeal croup.
- Exostosis; after injury.
- Aneurysm. Arterio sclerosis.
- Discharges turn grass green.
- Chronic synovitis; of knee joint.
- Encysted tumours at the back of wrist.
- Skin: cracked, dry, hard and of alabaster whiteness.

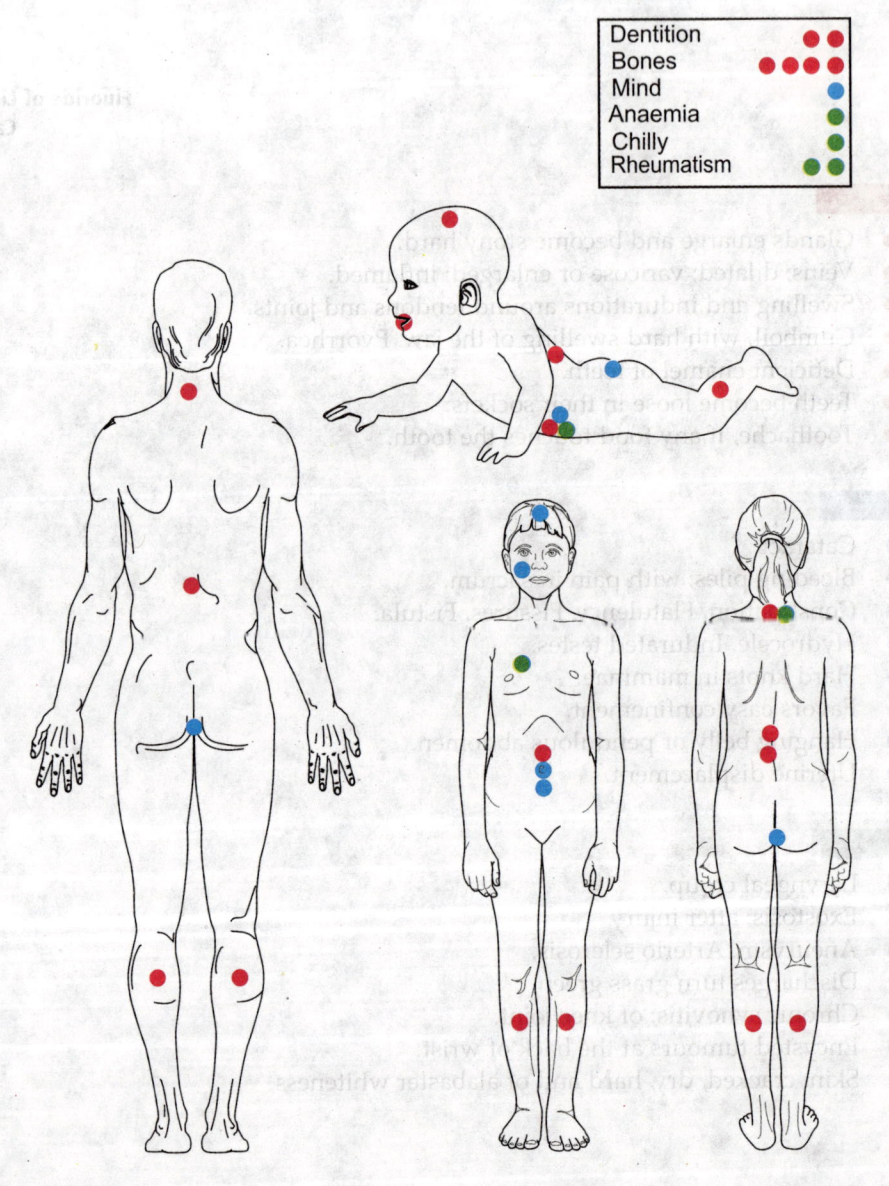

CALCAREA PHOSPHORICA

Phosphate of Lime
$Ca_3(PO_4)_2$

- For persons anemic and dark complexioned, dark hair and eyes; thin spare subjects, instead of fat.
- During first and second dentition of scrofulous children; delayed or complicated teething.
- Children; emaciated, unable to stand; slow in learning to walk; sunken, flabby abdomen.
- Malassimilation. Rickets.
- Cranial bones thin and brittle; fontanelles and sutures remain open too long, or close and re-open.
- Tendency of bones to soften or spine to curve.
- Spine weak, disposed to curvatures, especially to the left; unable to support body; neck weak, unable to support head.
- Non-union of bones; promotes callous.

- Feels complaints more when thinking about them.
- Girls at puberty, tall growing rapidly.
- Ailments of school girls: anemia, acne, vertex headache, diarrhea; dyspepsia,.
- At every attempt to eat, colicky pains in abdomen.
- Flatulent dyspepsia > by eating.
- Diarrhea and great flatulence during dentition.
- Fistula in ano, alternating with chest symptoms.

- Anemia, after acute diseases or chronic wasting diseases.
- Lack of animal heat; cold sweat and general coldness of body.
- Rheumatism of cold weather; getting well in spring and returning in autumn.
- Oozing of bloody fluid from navel of infants. Festering navel.
- Pain in chest and neck from drafts.

SURFACE MARKING OF KEYNOTES

CALCAREA SULPHURICA

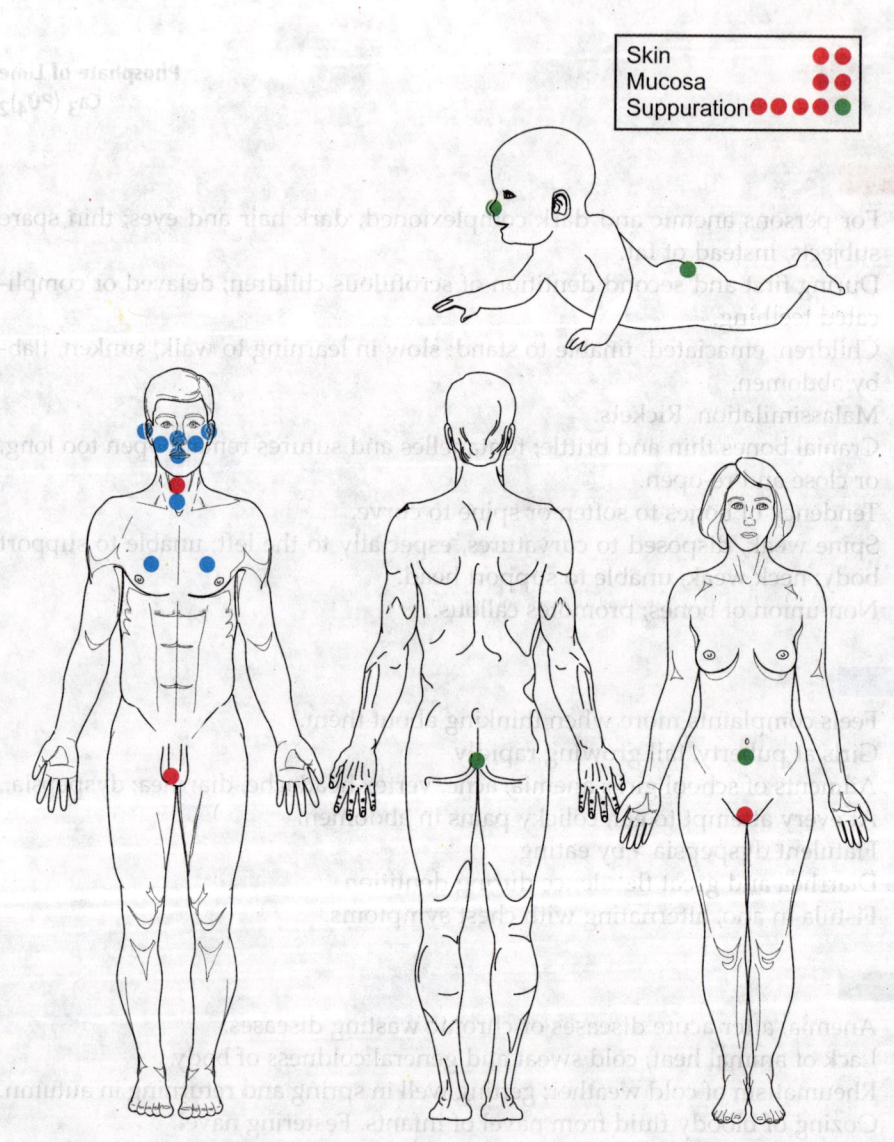

CALCAREA SULPHURICA

Sulphate of Lime
$CaSO_4 \cdot 2H_2O$

- Affects glands, mucous membranes, bones and skin.
- Mucous discharges in cough, leucorrhoea, gonorrhea etc., are yellow, thick and lumpy.
- Third stage of inflammation, with lumpy or bloody discharge.
- Tendency to suppuration, after pus has found its vent.
- Pus is thick, yellow, lumpy and bloody.
- Abscesses; to reduce and control suppurations.
- Cuts, wounds, bruises, etc. unhealthy, discharging pus; they do not heal readily.

- Pimples and pustules on the face.
- Suppurative otitis media. Ozaena. Gum-boils. Quinsy.
- Empyema.
- Third stage of bronchitis.

- Painful abscess about anus, in cases of fistula.
- Infants; with bloody coryza, diarrhea or eczema.
- To limit the discharge of pus from stitches after caesarean section.

SURFACE MARKING OF KEYNOTES

CALENDULA

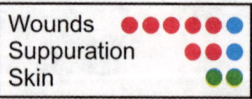
Wounds
Suppuration
Skin

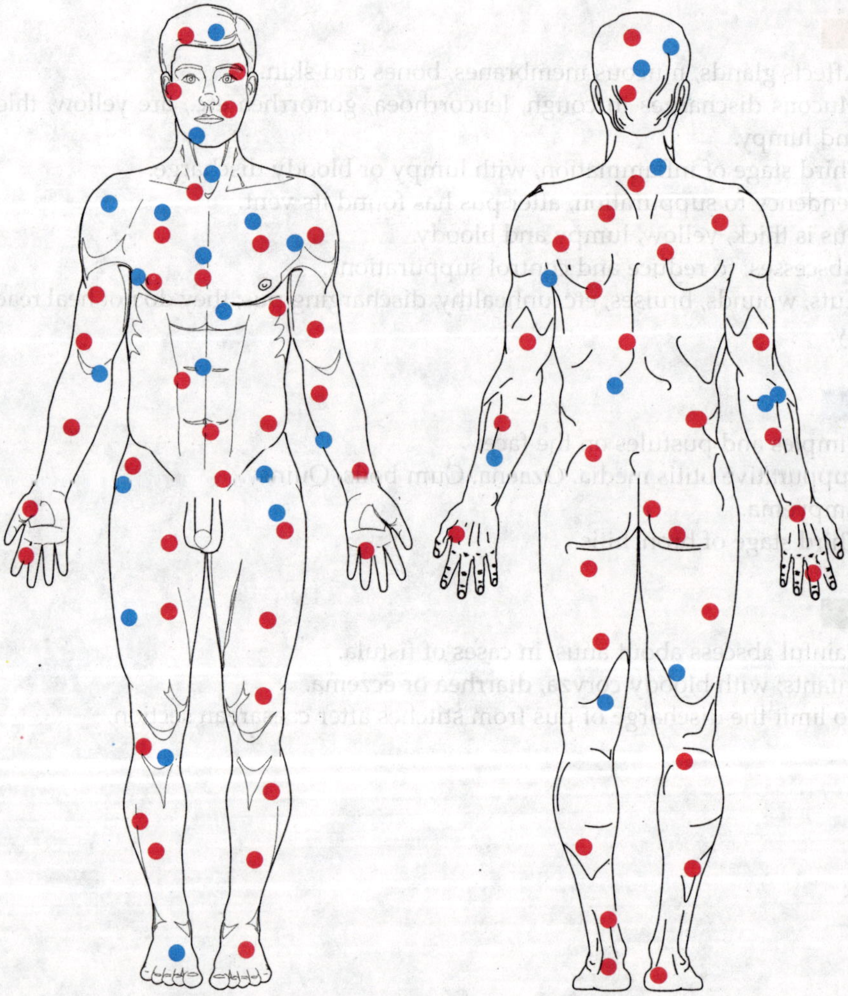

CALENDULA

Marigold
Compositae

- External wounds with or without loss of substance; torn and jagged looking wounds; post-surgical operations; to promote healthy granulation and prevent excessive suppuration and disfiguring scars.
- Calendula is almost specific for clean, surgical cuts or lacerated wounds, to prevent excessive suppuration.
- Rupture of muscles of tendons; lacerations during labor; wounds penetrating articulations with loss of synovial fluids.
- Traumatic affections: to secure union by first intention and prevent suppuration.
- In all cases of loss of soft parts when union cannot be effected by means of adhesive plaster.

- Wounds: with sudden pain during febrile heat.
- Old, neglected, offensive wound; threatening gangrene.
- Traumatic and idiopathic neuroma; neuritis from lacerated wound; exhausted from loss of blood and excessive pain.

- Constitutional tendency to erysipelas.
- Ulcers: irritable, inflamed, sloughing, varicose; painful as if beaten; excessive secretion of pus.
- Cancer, as an intercurrent remedy.

SURFACE MARKING OF KEYNOTES

CAMPHORA

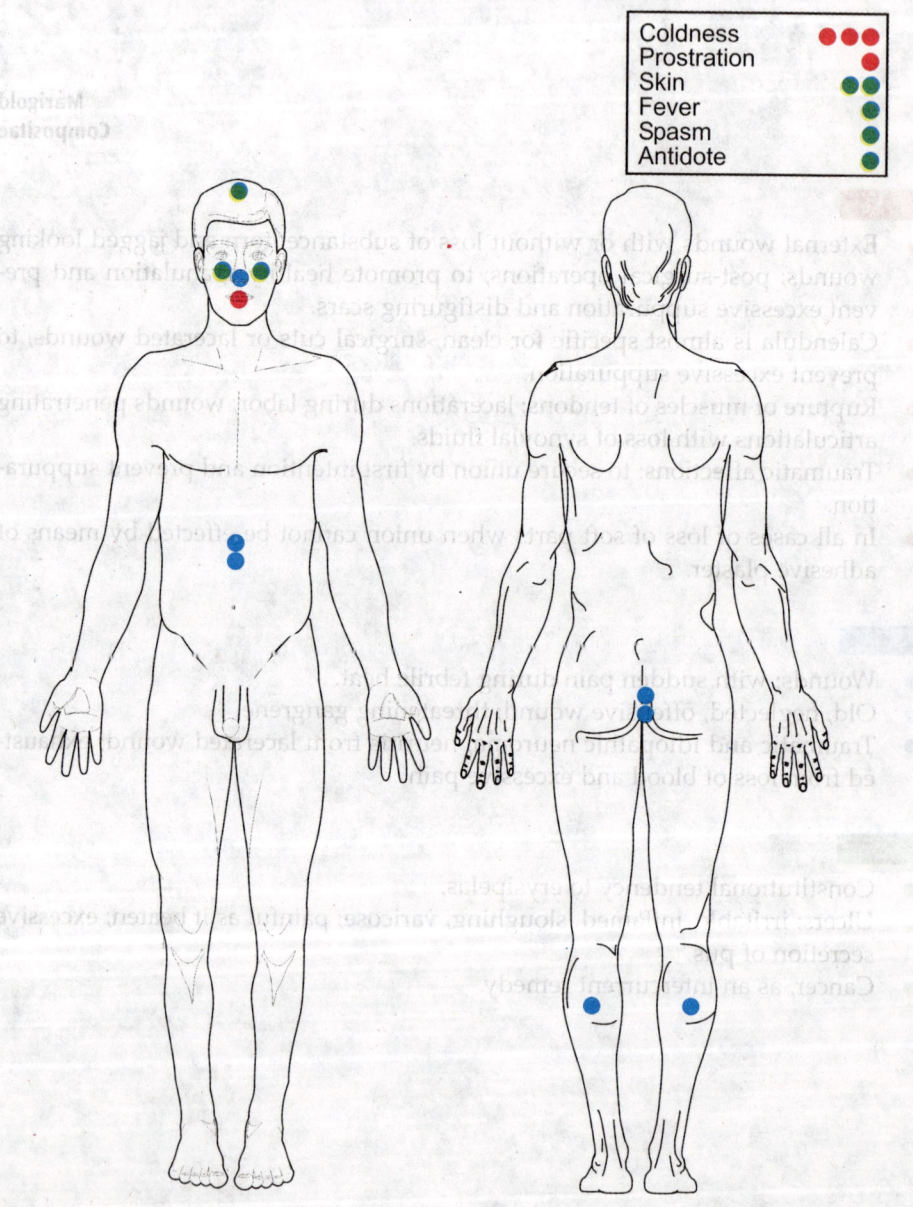

CAMPHORA

Camphor
Lauraceae

- Great coldness of the surface with sudden and complete prostration of the vital force.
- Surface cold to the touch, yet cannot bear to be covered; throws off all coverings.
- Exceedingly sensitive to cold air.
- Tongue cold, flabby, trembling.
- Entire body painfully sensitive to slightest touch.

- Pain better while thinking of it.
- In first stages of cholera morbus and Asiatic cholera; severe, long-lasting chill.
- Sudden attacks of vomiting and diarrhea; nose cold and pointed; anxious and restless; skin and breath cold.
- Cramps in calves.

- Measles and scarlatina when eruption does not appear; with pale or cold blue, hippocratic face; child will not be covered.
- All sequelae of measles.
- Often a remedy in congestive chill; pernicious, intermittent; pulse weak, externally small, scarcely perceptible.
- Tetanic spasms with showing of the teeth.
- Corrects spoiled cases and antidotes most of the medicines, especially from vegetable kingdom.

SURFACE MARKING OF KEYNOTES

CANTHARIDES

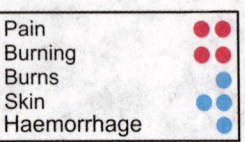

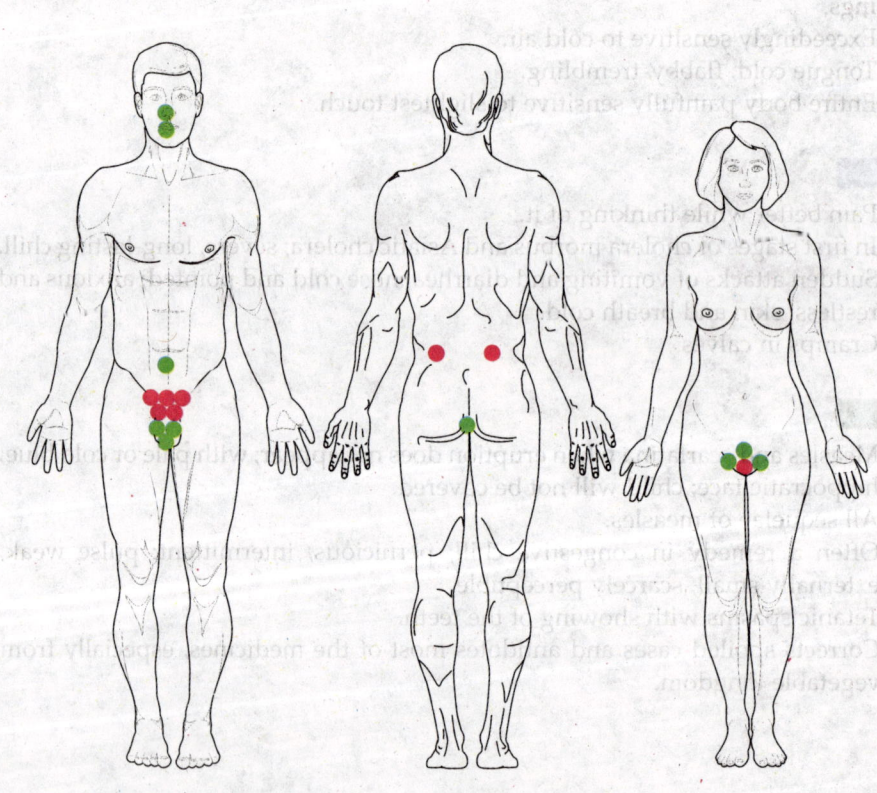

88 C

CANTHARIDES

Spanish Flies
Cantharideae

- Pain; raw, sore, burning in every part of body, internally and externally; with extreme weakness.
- Intolerable urging, before, during and after urination; violent pains in bladder.
- Constant urging to urinate, passing but a few drops at a time, which is mixed with blood.
- Burning, cutting pains in urethra during micturition; violent tenesmus and strangury.
- Acute nephritis; nephritic colic.
- Cystitis. Strangury.

- Burns and scalds, relieved by cold applications: burns before blisters form and when they have formed.
- Skin: vesicular erysipelas; turning black; vesicles all over body which are sore and suppurating.
- Erythema from exposure to sun's rays.

- Hemorrhages from nose, mouth, intestines, genital and urinary organs.
- Stool: passage of white or pale, red, tough mucus, like scrapings from the intestines, with streaks of blood, with tenesmus of rectum and bladder.
- Sexual desire; increased both sexes; not > by coitus; preventing sleep; violent priapism, with excessive pain.
- Bloody, nocturnal emission.
- Expels moles, dead foetus, placenta, promotes fecundity.

SURFACE MARKING OF KEYNOTES

CARBO VEGETABILIS

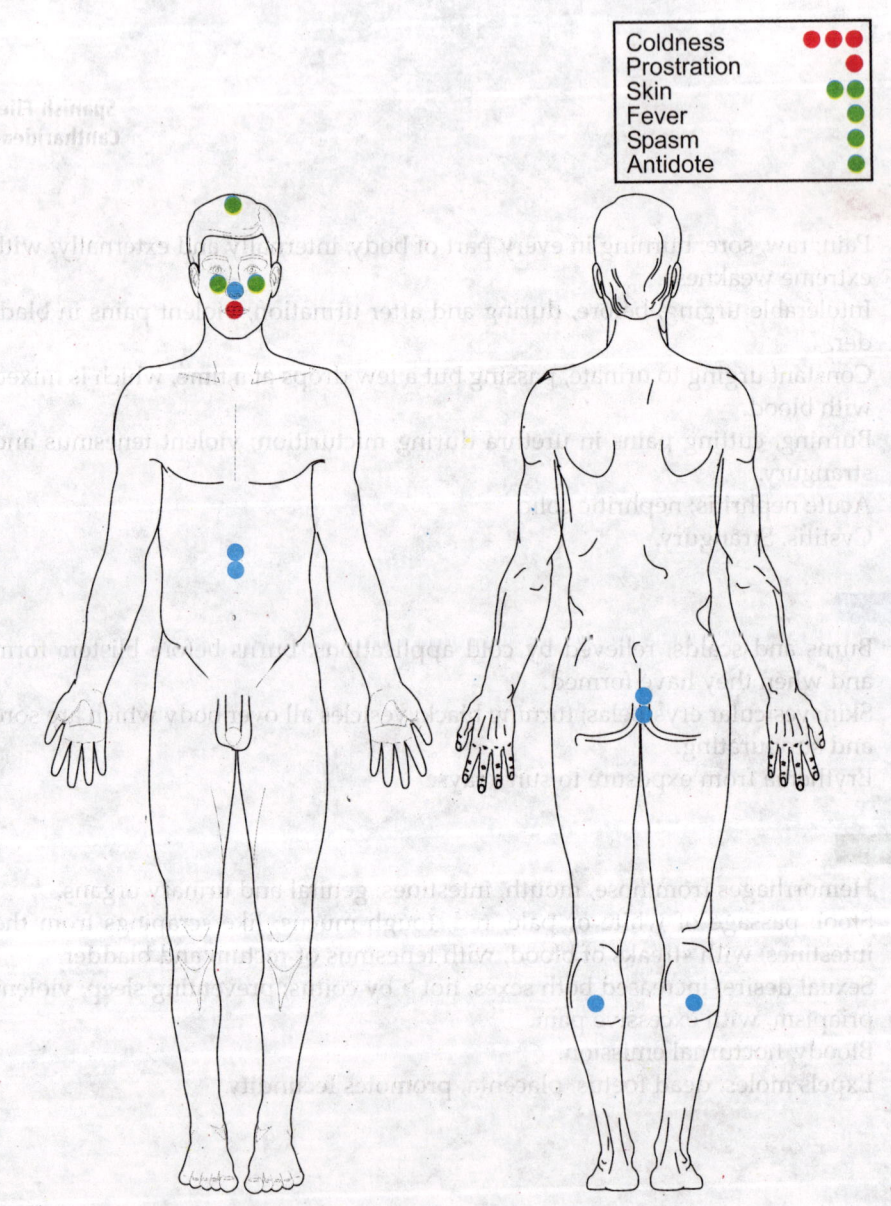

90 C

CARBO VEGETABILIS

Vegetable Charcoal
C(Impure)

- Fat, sluggish, lazy patients with a tendency to chronicity of complaints.
- Persons who have never fully recovered from the exhausting effects of some previous illness.
- Vital powers nearly exhausted from loss of vital fluids; from serious or grave diseases; from effects of drug (quinine, mercury) and disease (measles, pertussis, typhoid, intermittents, asthma; from obstinate complications.
- Desire to be constantly fanned.
- Weakness, flatulence, foetor or air hunger, are present with most of the complaints. Always weak, sick and exhausted.
- Weak digestion: simplest food disagrees; effects of a debauch, late suppers, rich food.
- Excessive accumulation of gas especially in upper abdomen < lying down; after eating or drinking, sensation as if stomach would burst.
- Eructations give temporary relief.
- Frequent, involuntary, cadaverous-smelling stools, followed by burning.

- Hemorrhages; from any mucus outlet; blood dark, oozing, from shock, after surgical operations, persistent for hours or days.
- Epistaxis in daily attacks; < exertion; with pale face.
- Looseness of teeth, easily bleeding gums.
- Diseases of the venous systems predominate; symptoms of imperfect oxidation. Venous stasis.
- Deficient capillary circulation causes blueness of skin and coldness of extremities.

- Hippocratic face; very pale, cold with cold sweat.
- Asthma: in aged, with blue skin; > summer.
- Hoarseness: < evenings; damp evening air; warm, wet weather.
- In the last stages of disease, with copious cold sweat, cold breath, cold tongue, voice lost, this remedy may save a life.
- Awakens often from cold limbs and suffers from cold knees at night.
- Senile gangrene of fingers and toes.
- Ulcers; foul, burning, varicose and bleeding.
- Septic conditions.

SURFACE MARKING OF KEYNOTES

CAUSTICUM

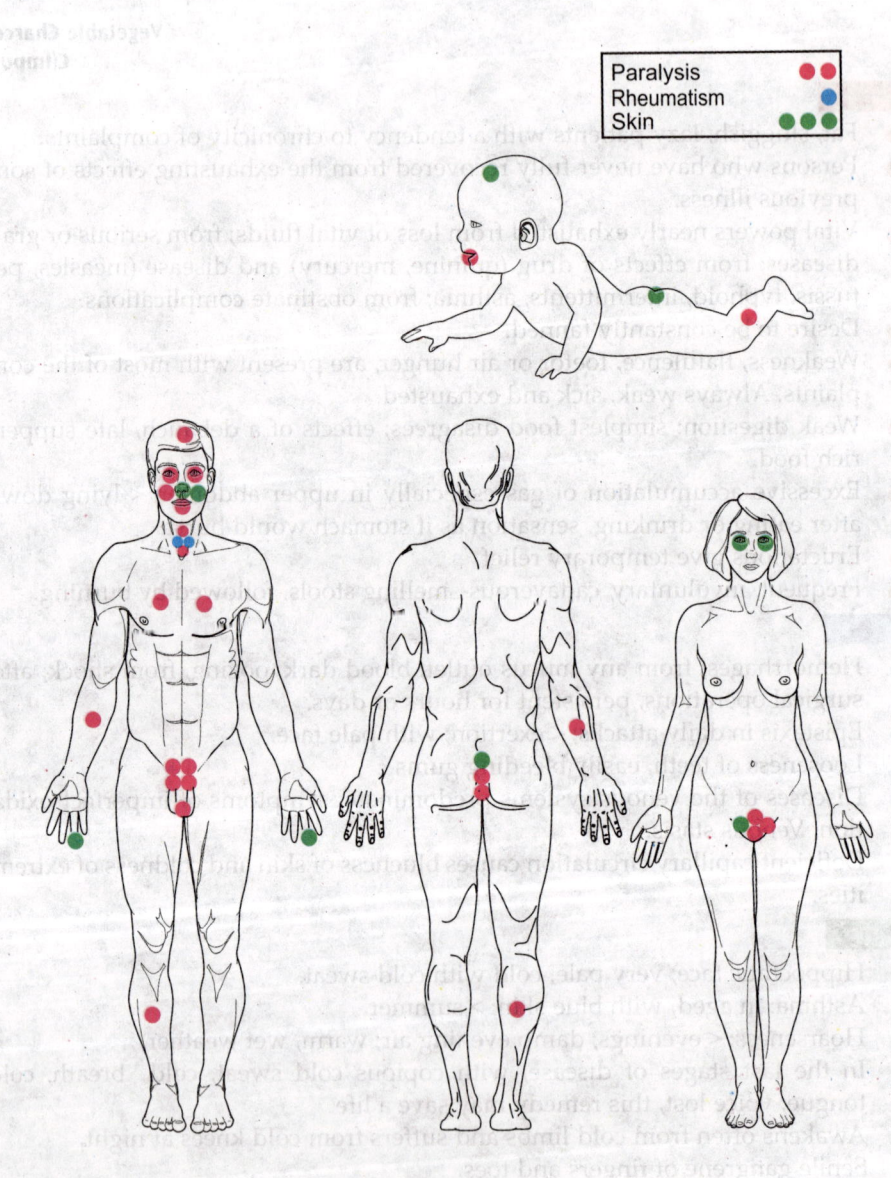

92 C

CAUSTICUM

Tinctura acris sine kali
Potassium Hydrate

- Adapted to persons with dark hair and rigid fiber; weakly, psoric, with excessively yellow, sallow complexion.
- Children slow in learning to walk and talk.
- Rawness or soreness: of scalp, throat, respiratory tract, rectum, anus, urethra, vagina, uterus.
- Paralysis: of single parts; vocal organs, tongue, eyelids, face, extremities, bladder; generally, of right side; from exposure to cold wind or draft; after typhoid, typhus or diphtheria; from lead; gradually appearing.
- Drooping of upper eyelids; cannot keep them open.
- Urine involuntary: when coughing, sneezing, blowing the nose.
- Retention of urine: after labor, after surgical operations.
- Urine; dribbles or passes slowly; passed better on sitting.

- Chronic rheumatic affections, with contraction of the flexor and deformities or stiffness of the joints; tension and shortening of muscles.
- Cough: with rawness and soreness in chest; with inability to expectorate; > drinking cold water; on expiration; with pain in hips; remaining after pertussis.
- Hoarseness with rawness, and aphonia < in the morning.

- Skin prone to intertrigo during dentition or convulsions with eruption of teeth.
- Cicatrices, especially deep burns, scalds, freshen up, become sore again.
- Warts: large, jagged, often pedunculated; bleeding easily; exuding moisture; small, all over the body; on eyelids, face, nose, tip of fingers.
- Constipation: frequent, ineffectual desire; stool passes better while standing; tough and shining; in children with nocturnal enuresis.
- Menses: too early; too feeble; only during the day; cease on lying down.

SURFACE MARKING OF KEYNOTES

CHAMOMILLA

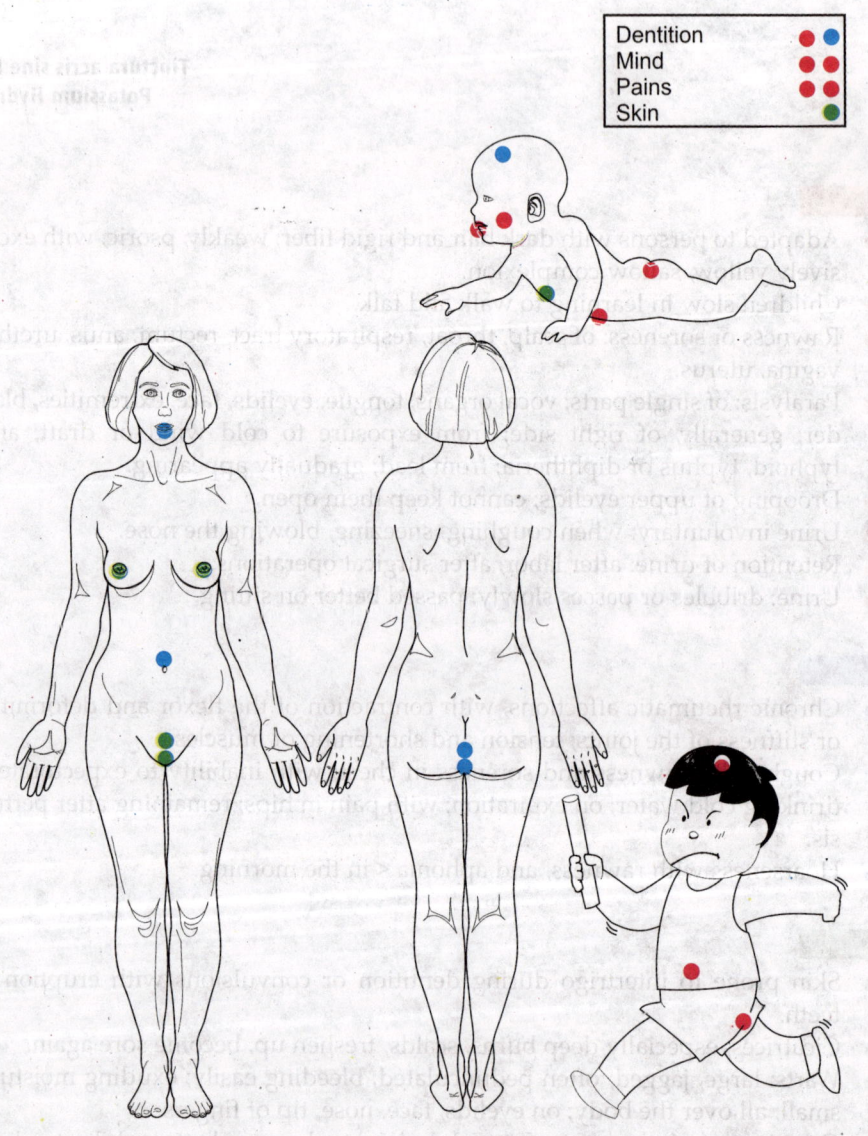

CHAMOMILLA

Matricaria Chamomilla
Compositae

- Children, new-born and during period of dentition.
- Child exceedingly irritable, fretful; quiet only when carried; impatient, wants this or that and becomes angry when refused, or when offered, petulantly rejects it.
- Complaint from anger, especially chill, fever, colic, diarrhea, jaundice, and convulsions.
- Pain; seems unendurable, drives to despair; with heat, hot sweat, thirst, fainting and numbness of affected part; < by heat, evening before midnight, eructations.
- *Cham.* is *Opium* of Homeopathy.
- One cheek red and hot, the other pale and cold.

- Convulsions of children from nursing, after a fit of anger in mother.
- Toothache; < after warm drinks, on entering warm room, in bed, from coffee, during menses or pregnancy.
- Spells of colic, < night, after anger, urinating, > warm applications.
- Diarrhea: from cold, anger or chagrin; during dentition; after tobacco; in child-bed; from downward motion.
- Stool green, watery, corroding, like chopped eggs and spinach; hot, very offensive, like rotten eggs.

- Labor pains: spasmodic, distressing, wants to get away from them; tearing down the legs; press upward.
- Breasts sore, nipples inflamed, tender to touch; infants breasts tender.
- Membranous dysmenorrhoea, especially at puberty.
- Rash of infants and of nursing mothers.

SURFACE MARKING OF KEYNOTES

CHELIDONIUM MAJUS

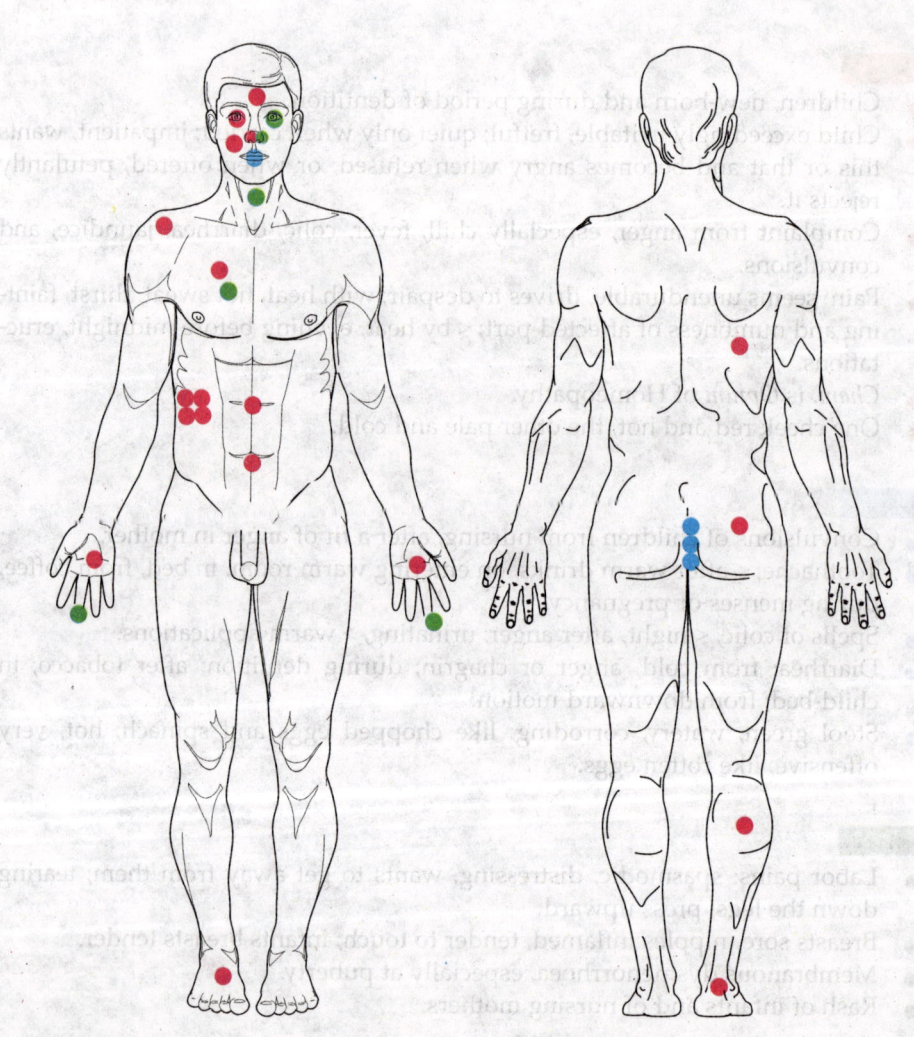

96 C

CHELIDONIUM MAJUS

Celandine
Papoveraceae

- Persons subject to hepatic, gastric and abdominal complaints; every age, sex and temperament.
- Affects right side most; right eye, right lung, right hypochondrium and abdomen, right hip and leg; right foot cold as ice, left natural.
- Face, forehead, nose, cheeks remarkably yellow.
- Yellow-gray colour of the skin; wilted skin; of the palms of hands.
- Constant pain under the lower and inner angle of right scapula.
- Hepatic diseases; jaundice, pain in right shoulder.
- Gall stones, with pain under the right shoulder-blade.

- Tongue coated thickly yellow, with red edges showing imprint of teeth.
- Constipation: stool, hard, round balls like sheep's dung.
- Alternate constipation and diarhea.
- Diarrhea: at night; slimy, light-gray; bright-yellowish; brown or white, watery, pasty; involuntary.

- Periodic orbital neuralgia, with excessive lachrymation; tears fairly gush out.
- Cough: as from dust; with much rattling; but little expectoration, or it flies from mouth.
- Pneumonia of right lung; liver complications.
- Flapping of the alae nasi.
- Cold finger tips.

SURFACE MARKING OF KEYNOTES

CINA

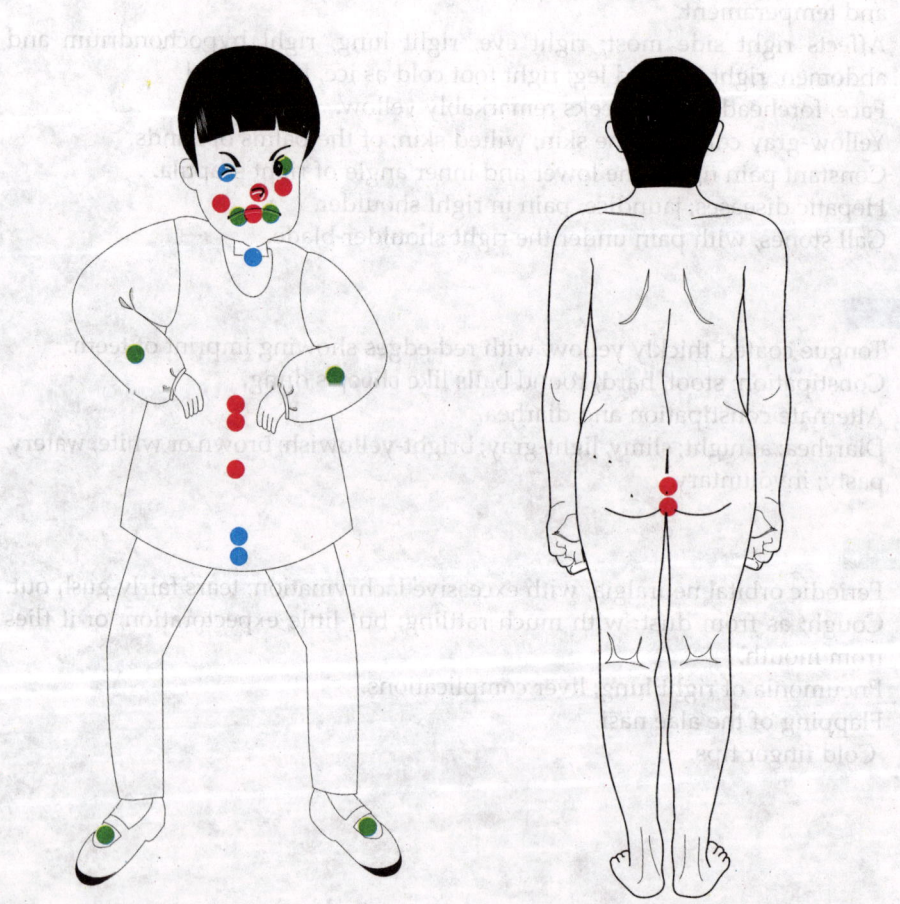

98 C

CINA

Worm seed
Compositae

- Adapted to children, who are big, fat, rosy and scrofulous, with dark hair; very touchy, ugly, cross, petulant and dissatisfied.
- Does not want to be touch, wants to be rocked.
- Children, suffering from worms; pitiful weeping when awake, starts and screams during sleep; grinding of teeth at night; ascarides.
- Face is pale; sickly white and bluish appearance around mouth; sickly, with dark rings under the eyes.
- One cheek red, the other pale.
- Constantly digging and boring at the nose; picks the nose all the time; itching of nose; rubs nose on pillow, or shoulder of nurse.
- Canine hunger: hungry soon after a full meal; after vomiting; alternating with loss of appetite; before chill or follows sweat, in paraplegia.
- Craving for sweets and different things; refuses mother's milk.
- Twisting, cutting, pinching abdominal pain from worms, > pressure.
- Itching at anus.

- Weak sight, from masturbation.
- Cough; dry with sneezing; spasmodic, gagging in the morning; periodic; returning spring and fall; < speaking or moving.
- Urine: turbid when passed, turns milky and semisolid after standing.
- Bed wetting < every full moon.

- Clean tongue; with vomiting; during fever.
- Spasms; squint; due to worms.
- Children tosses arms from side to side, stretches out feet spasmodically.
- Complaints concomitant to yawning, which comes on whenever someone yawns.

SURFACE MARKING OF KEYNOTES

CINCHONA OFFICINALIS

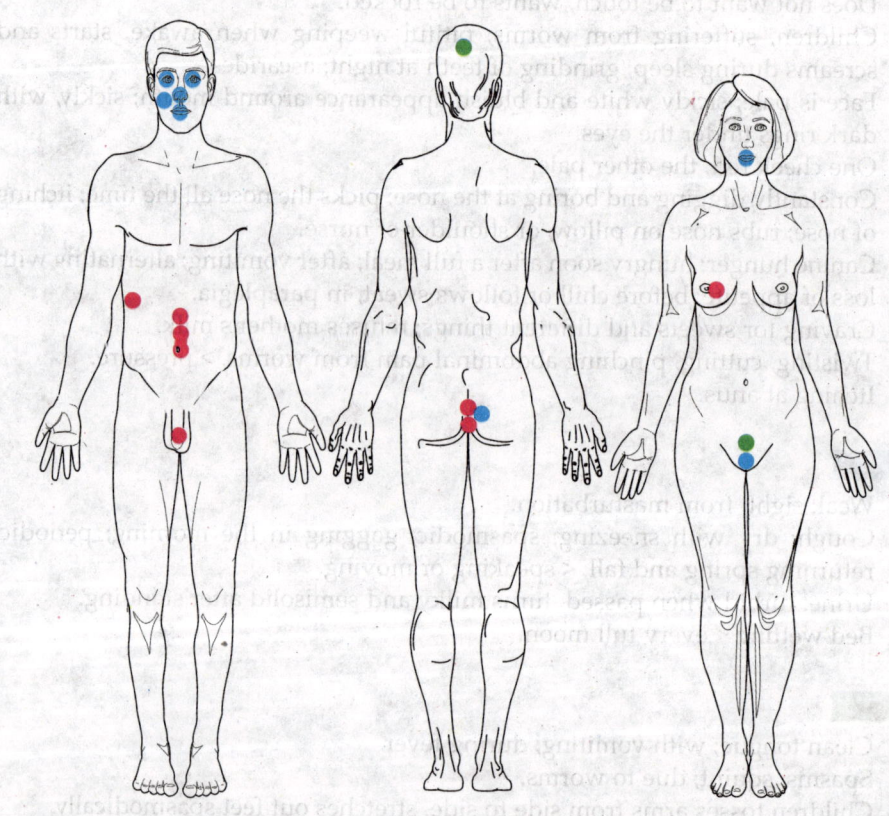

100 C

CINCHONA OFFICINALIS

Peruvian Bark
Rubiaceae

- Apathetic, indifferent, taciturn, despondent, gloomy.
- Ailments; from loss of vital fluids, especially hemorrhages, excessive lactation, diarrhea, suppuration, of malarial origin, with marked periodicity; return every other day.
- Great debility, trembling, aversion to exercise; entire nervous system extremely sensitive.
- Excessive flatulence of stomach and bowels or whole abdomen; fermentation, borborygmus; post operative gas pains, belching gives no relief.
- Colic: periodical, at a certain hour each day; < at night, after eating; > bending double.
- Gall stone colic. Jaundice.
- Stools: lienteric; dark, foul; watery; bloody; painless; < eating; at night, from fruits; milk, bear, during hot weather.

- Face pale, sickly, hippocratic; eyes sunken and surrounded by blue margins.
- Toothache while nursing the child, > by pressing teeth firmly, warmth.
- Intermittent fever; returns every 7 or 14 days; never at night; stages of chill, heat and sweat well marked; chill, then thirst, then heat, then thirst; drenching sweats; at night; < least motion.
- Disposition to hemorrhage; from every orifice of the body; from mouth, nose, bowels or uterus; long continued.

- Pains: drawing or tearing; in every joint, all the bones; < by slightest touch, but > by hard pressure.
- Headache; bursting, throbbing, anemic; after hemorrhage or sexual excesses; from occiput over whole head; < sitting or lying, must stand or walk.
- Menses; too early, dark, profuse, clotted, with abdominal distention.
- Bad effects from excessive tea drinking.

SURFACE MARKING OF KEYNOTES

COLCHICUM AUTUMNALE

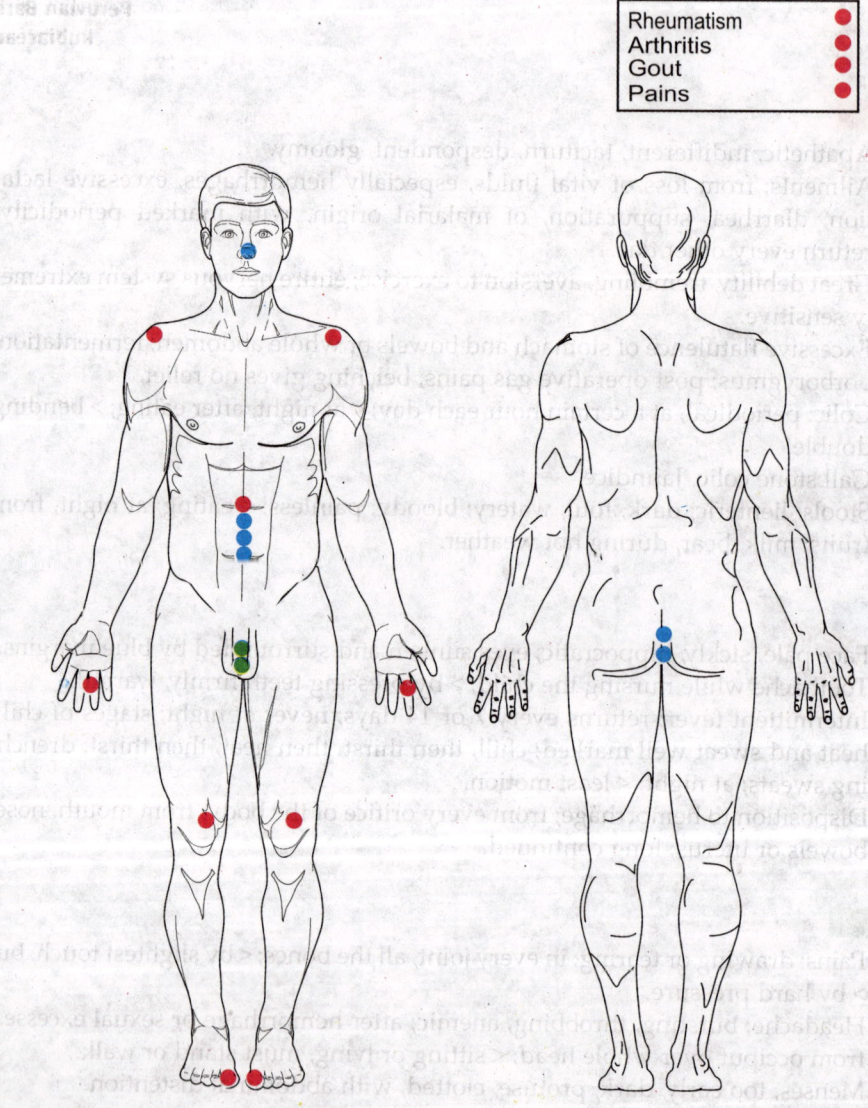

Rheumatism	●
Arthritis	●
Gout	●
Pains	●

COLCHICUM AUTUMNALE

Meadow saffron
Liliaceae

- Adapted to the rheumatic; gouty diathesis; persons of robust vigorous constitution; diseases of old people.
- Arthritic pains in joints; patient screams with pain on touching a joint or stubbing a toe; joints red hot swollen and stiff.
- Pains are drawing, tearing, pressing; light or superficial during warm weather; affect the bones and deeper tissues, when air is cold; pains go from left to right.
- Affected parts very sensitive to contact and motion.
- External impressions, light, noise, strong odors, contact, bad manners, make him almost beside himself.
- Aversion to food; loathing even the sight or still more the smell of it.

- Smell, painfully acute; nausea and faintness from the odor of cooking food, especially fish; eggs or fat meat.
- Autumnal dysentery, discharges contain white mucus and "scrapings of intestines".
- Stools; very painful, offensive, choleric; of shreddy, bloody, gelatinous, mucus.
- The abdomen is immensely distended with gas, contracts when touched.
- Burning, or icy coldness in stomach and abdomen.

- Urine: dark, scanty or suppressed; in drops, with white sediment; bloody, brown, black, inky.
- Urine contains clots of putrid decomposed blood, albumin, sugar.

SURFACE MARKING OF KEYNOTES

COLOCYNTHIS

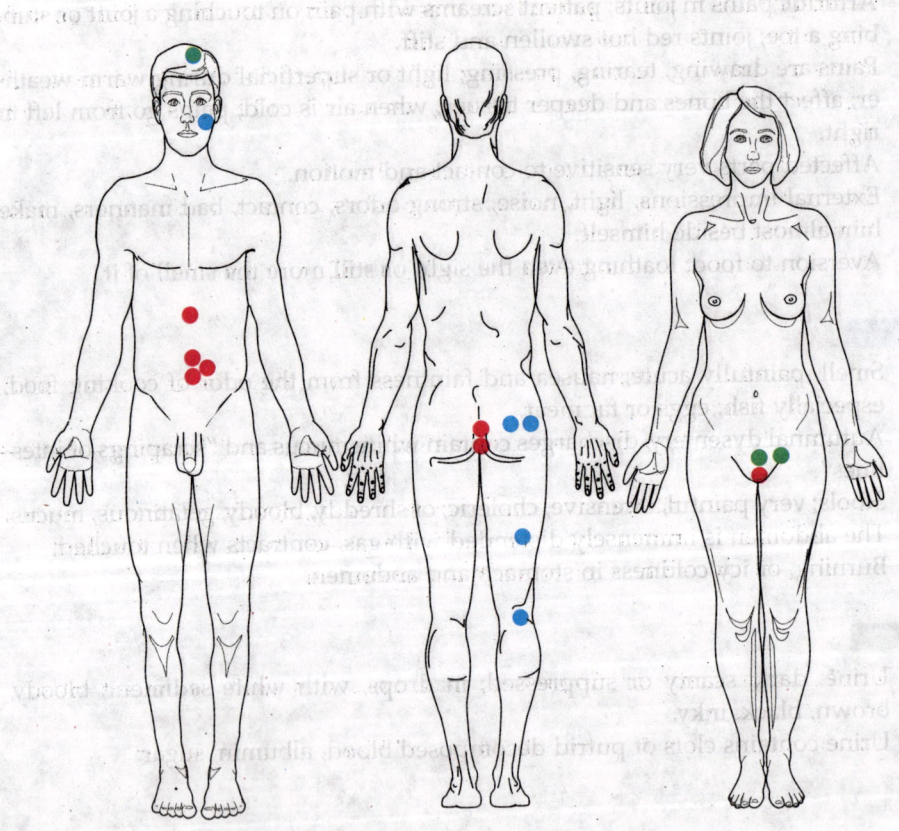

Mind	●

104 C

COLOCYNTHIS

Squirting Cucumber
Cucurbitaceae

- Affections from anger, with indignation, particularly colic, vomiting, diarrhea and suppression of menses.
- Agonizing pain in abdomen causing patient to bend double, with restlessness, twisting and turning to obtain relief > by hard pressure worse after eating or drinking.
- Intestines feel squeezed between stones.
- Stools; frothy, watery, shreddy, yellow, sourish or gelatinous; with flatulence and pain.

- Prosopalgia, with eye symptoms, or alternating, with pain in celiac region, with chilliness.
- Crampy pain in hip, as though screwed in a vise, > lies upon affected side.
- Sciatica: shooting pain, like lightning-shocks, down the whole limb, left hip, left thigh, left knee, into popliteal fossa; > pressure, heat; < least motion, rotation, at night.

- Vertigo: when quickly turning head, especially to the left, as if he would fall; from stimulants.
- Dysmenorrhoea, < eating and drinking.
- Ovarian cyst, with pain > flexing thigh on pelvis.

SURFACE MARKING OF KEYNOTES

CONIUM MACULATUM

Scrofulous	🔴🔴
Cancer	🔴
Injuries	🔴🔴🔴
Paralysis	🔴
Sweat	🟢

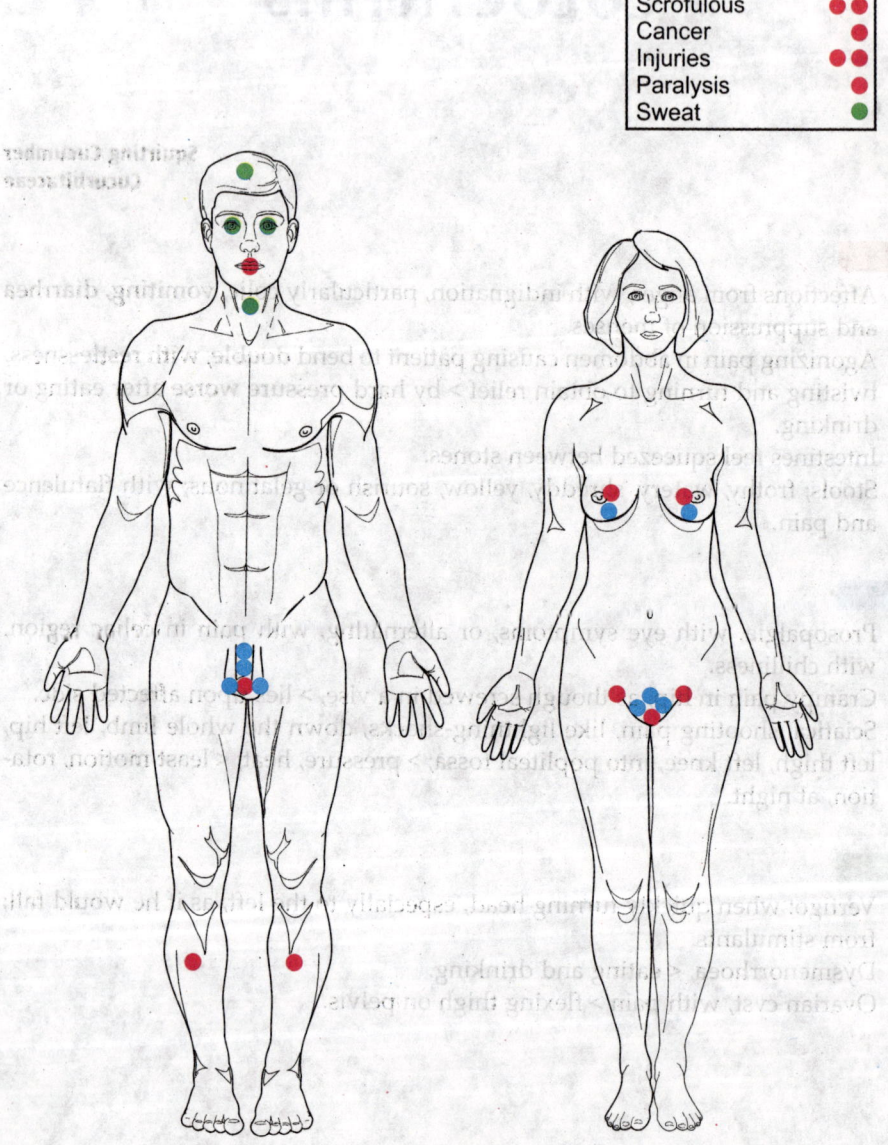

CONIUM MACULATUM

Poison Hemlock
Umbelliferae

- Especially for diseases of old men, old maids, old bachelors; with rigid muscular fibre; cancerous and scrofulous persons with enlarged glands.
- Glandular induration of stony hardness; of mammae and ovary in persons of cancerous tendency; after bruises and injuries of glands.
- Ill effects of contusions, blows, fall; overstraining, over work.
- Bad effects: of suppressed sexual desire, or from excessive indulgence, or suppressed menses.
- Incordination, paralysis, trembling, uncertain gait, difficult speech, progressive debility.

- Breasts sore, hard and painful before and during menstruation.
- Menses: feeble, suppressed, too late, scanty, of short duration; with red pimples over body; stopped by taking cold; by putting hands in cold water.
- Leucorrhoea: ten days after menses; acrid; bloody; milky; profuse; thick; intermits.
- Stony, hard induration of the testicles. Impotence. Spermatorrhea.
- Great difficulty in voiding urine; flow intermits, then flows again; > standing; prostatic or uterine affections.

- Vertigo: especially when lying down or turning in bed; moving the head slightly, or even the eyes; on turning the head to the left; of old people.
- Photophobia and excessive lachrymation; without inflammation, < using eyes in artificial light.
- Cataract after eye injury.
- Cough; in spasmodic paroxysm caused by dry spot in larynx; worse at night, when lying down, and during pregnancy.
- Sweat day and night, as soon as one sleeps, or even when closing the eyes.

SURFACE MARKING OF KEYNOTES

DIGITALIS PURPUREA

 Dropsy

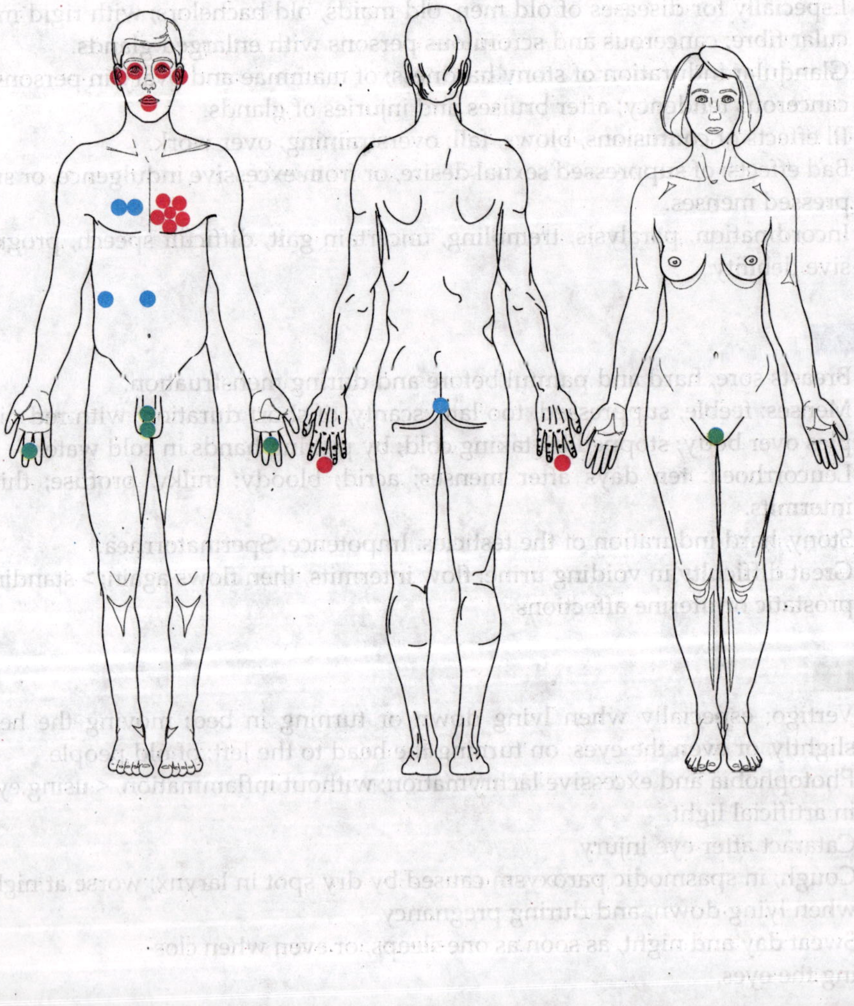

108 D

DIGITALIS PURPUREA

Foxglove
Scrophulariaceae

- Weak heart without valvular complications.
- Hypertrophy with dilatation of heart.
- Attacks of angina < raising arms.
- Sensation as if heart would stop beating if she moved.
- Pulse full, irregular, very slow and weak; intermitting every third, fifth or seventh beat.
- Blueness of skin, eyelids, lips, tongue, nails, cyanosis.
- Distended veins on lids, ears, lips and tongue.
- Fatal syncope may occur when being raised to upright position.
- Dropsy: post-scarlatinal; in brights's disease; with suppression of urine; of internal and external parts; with fainting when there are organic affections of the heart.

- Great weakness of chest, cannot bear to talk.
- Respiration irregular, difficult, deep sighing.
- Deathly nausea not > by vomiting or with faint sinking at the pit of the stomach, exhaustion, extreme prostration; feels as if he were dying.
- Liver, enlarged, sore, hard, painful. Jaundice.
- Stools: very light, ash-colored; delayed, chalky; almost white; pipestem stool; involuntary.

- Sudden flushes of heat, followed by great nervous weakness and irregular intermitting pulse, occurring at the climacteric; < by least motion.
- Nightly emissions, with great weakness of genitals after coitus.
- Gonorrhea; balanitis, with oedema of prepuce.
- The fingers "go to sleep" frequently and easily.

SURFACE MARKING OF KEYNOTES

DROSERA ROTUNDIFOLIA

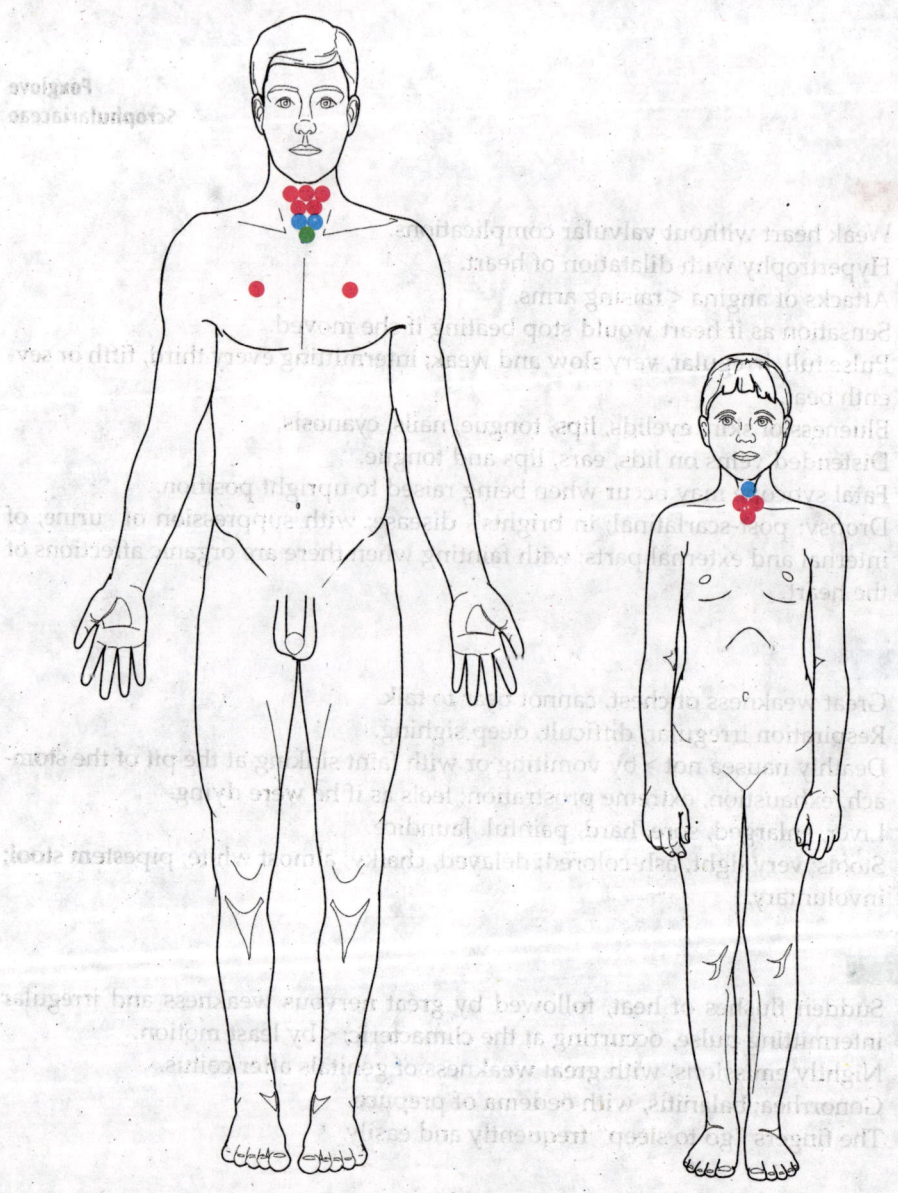

110 D

DROSERA ROTUNDIFOLIA

Sundew
Drosceracae

- Diseases prevailing during epidemic pertusis.
- Whooping-cough with violent paroxyma which follow each other rapidly, is scarcely able to get breath.
- Deep sounding, hoarse barking cough, < after midnight, during or after measles; spasmodic; with gagging, retching and vomiting.
- During cough; vomiting of water; mucus, and often bleeding from the nose and mouth.
- Cough: < by warmth, drinking, singing, laughing, weeping, lying down, after midnight.
- Constant, titillating cough in children, begins as soon as head touches pillow at night.
- Nocturnal cough of young persons in phthisis; bloody or purulent sputa.
- Tuberculosis of the lungs, larynx and bones; joints.

- Sensation of feather in larynx, exciting cough.
- Laryngeal phthisis following whooping-cough.
- Constriction and crawling in larynx; hoarseness, and yellow or green sputa.

- Clergyman's sore throat; with rough, scraping, dry sensation deep in the fauces; voice hoarse, deep, toneless, cracked, requires exertion to speak.

SURFACE MARKING OF KEYNOTES

DULCAMARA

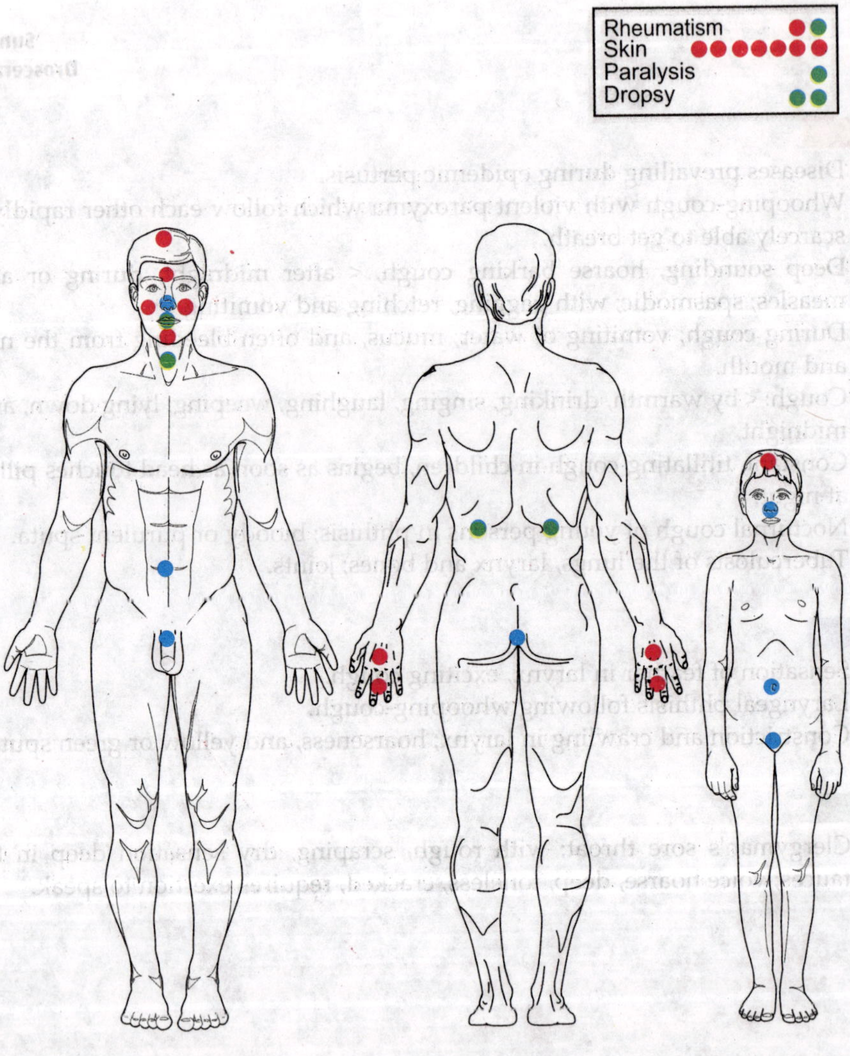

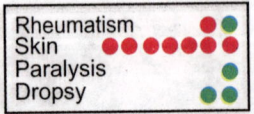

112 D

DULCAMARA

Bitter-sweat
Solanaceae

- Catarrhal rheumatism or skin affections, brought on or aggravated by exposure to cold, damp, rainy weather, or sudden changes in hot weather.
- Skin is delicate, sensitive to cold, liable to eruptions, especially urticaria.
- Urticaria over whole body, no fever; itching burns after scratching, < in warmth, sour stomach, > in cold.
- Eruptions, scaly, thick, crusty, moist, bleeding or herpetic.
- Thick brown-yellow crusts on scalp, face, forehead, temples, chin; with reddish borders, bleeding when scratched.
- Rash; before the menses; in new born.
- Ringworm, in the hair; in children.
- Warts, fleshy, large, smooth; on face or back of hands and fingers.

- Nose stuffs up in cold rain.
- Summer colds: with diarrhea.
- Cutting pains at navel followed by painful, green, slimy stools.
- Diarrhea, sour watery stools, < night, summer, damp cold weather, change from warm to cold weather.
- Catarrhal ischuria in grown-up children, with milky urine; from walking with bare feet in cold water.
- Involuntary urination from paralysis of bladder.

- Stiffness, numbness, aching and soreness of muscles on every exposure to cold especially of back and lions.
- Paralytic effects of single parts; vocal cords, tongue etc. Paralysed parts icy cold.
- Anasarca; after ague, rheumatism, scarlet fever.
- Dropsy: after suppressed sweat; suppressed eruptions; exposure to cold.

SURFACE MARKING OF KEYNOTES

EUPHRASIA

Injuries ●

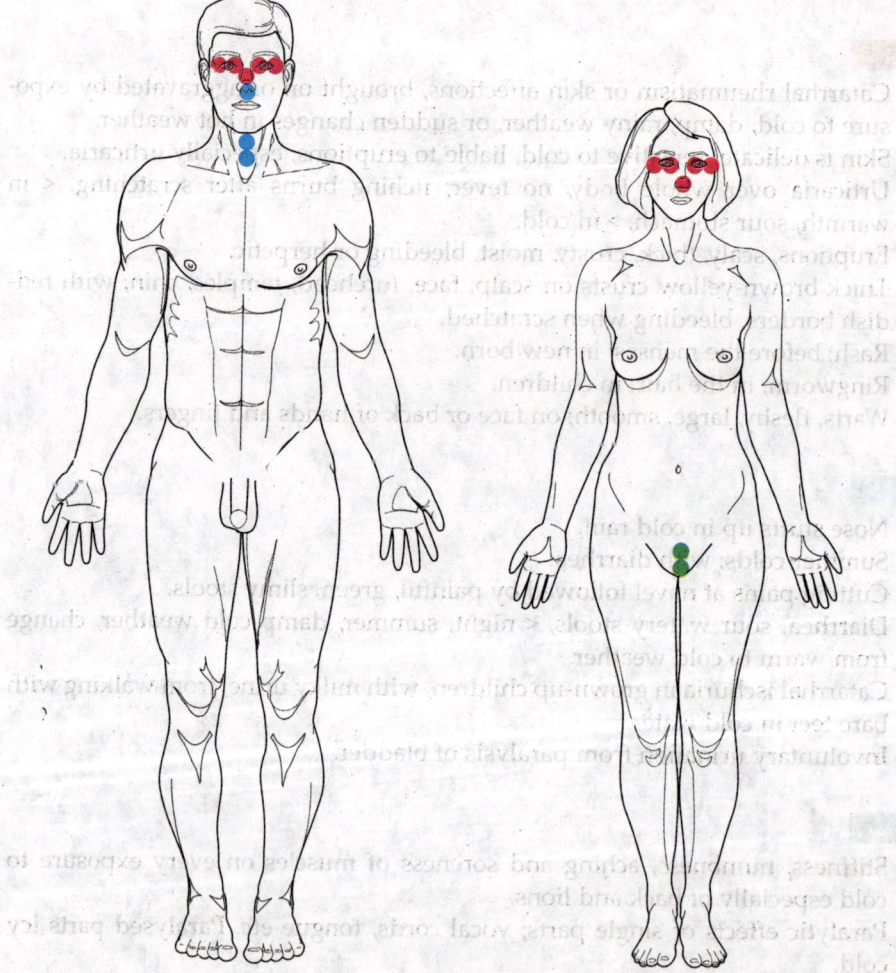

EUPHRASIA

Eye bright
Scrophularaceae

🔴

- Catarrhal affections of mucous membranes, especially of the eyes and nose.
- Profuse acrid lachrymation, with profuse, bland coryza.
- Profuse hot or acrid tears < open air, lying or coughing; leaving a varnish like mark.
- The eyes water all the time and are agglutinated in the morning; margins of lids red, swollen, burning.
- Conjunctivitis, with violent injection; of measles; instead of menses.

🔵

- Profuse bland fluent coryza; with cough and much expectoration, less when lying down, < from exposure to warm south wind.
- When attempting to clear the throat of an offensive mucus in the morning; gagging until he vomits the breakfast just eaten.
- Pertussis: excessive lachrymation during cough; cough only in day time.

🟢

- Menses: painful, regular, now lasting only one hour; or late, scanty, short, lasting only one day.
- Amenorrhoea, with ophthalmia and ulcer on right side of the nose.
- Bad effects from falls, contusions or mechanical injuries of external parts.

SURFACE MARKING OF KEYNOTES

FERRUM METALLICUM

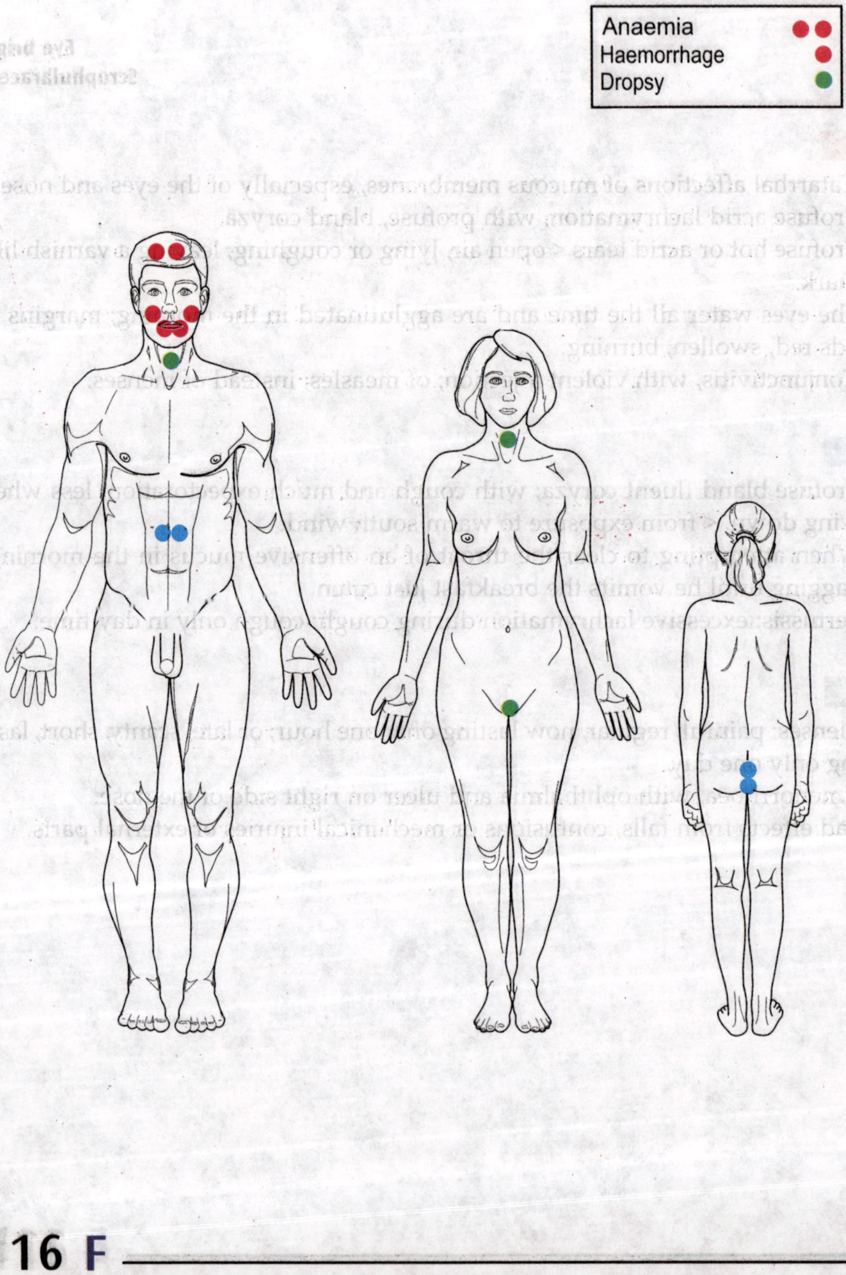

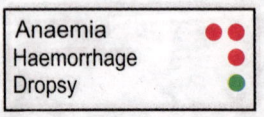

FERRUM METALLICUM

Iron
Fe

- It is adapted to young; anemic; pseudo-plethoric persons, who though looking strong are so weak that they are unable even to speak or walk, want to lie down, always feels better by walking slowly about.
- Extreme paleness of the face, lips and mucous membranes which become red and flushed on the least pain, emotion or exertion. Blushing.
- Red parts become white; face, lips, tongue and mucous membrane of mouth.
- Hemorrhagic diathesis; blood bright red, coagulates easily.
- Vertigo: < rising suddenly, on crossing the bridge, over water, on seeing flowing water.
- Throbbing; hammering headache, starts in the temples, extending to occiput, < cough, stooping, descending stairs; > letting hair down, lying down; with aversion to eating or drinking.

- Regurgitation and eructation of food in mouthfuls without nausea.
- Vomiting: immediately after midnight; of ingesta, as soon as food is eaten, leaves table suddenly and with one effort vomits everything eaten, can sit down and eat again; sour, acid; during pregnancy.
- Diarrhea: undigested stools at night, or while eating or drinking; painless with a good appetite; of consumptives.
- Constipation: from intestinal atony; ineffectual urging; stools hard, difficult, followed by backache or cramping pain in rectum; prolapsus recti of children, itching of anus at night due to ascarides.

- Dropsy: after loss of vital fluids; hemorrhages; abuse of quinine; suppressed intermittent.
- Exophthalmic goiter, after suppression of menses.
- Cough only in the day time, > by lying down, by eating.
- Menses: pale, watery, debilitating, too early, too profuse, protracted; intermit two or three days and then return; with labor like pains.

SURFACE MARKING OF KEYNOTES

FERRUM PHOSPHORICUM

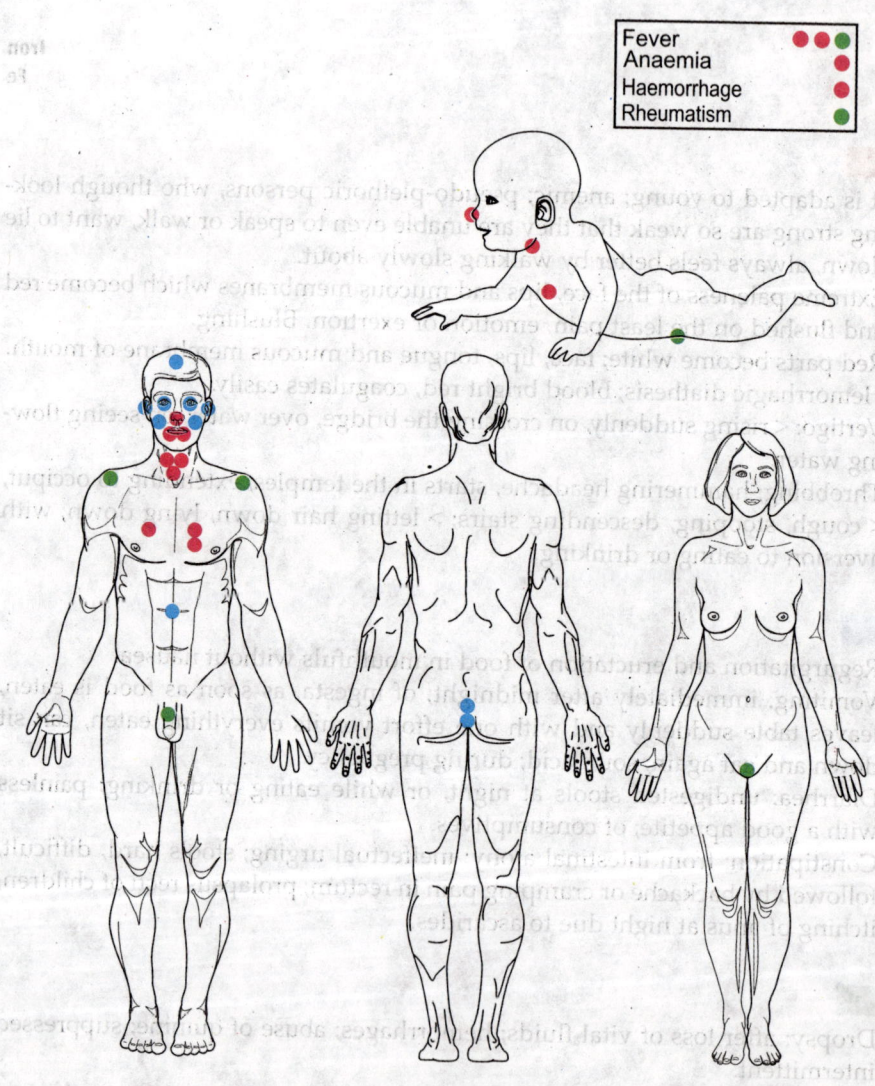

Fever	🔴🔴🟢
Anaemia	🔵
Haemorrhage	🔴
Rheumatism	🟢

118 F

FERRUM PHOSPHORICUM

Iron Phosphate
$Fe_3(PO_4)_2 \cdot 8H_2O$

- Initial stage of fever and inflammation especially before exudation commences.
- Local passive congestions and hemorrhages due to hyperaemia.
- Ill effects of checked sweat; mechanical injuries.
- Predisposition to catch cold.
- Epistaxis; bright red blood; in children.
- Sore throat, dry, red, inflamed, with much pain.
- Tonsils red and swollen.
- Laryngitis; with hoarseness; of singers.
- Acute exacerbation of tuberculosis.
- Acute, febrile or initial stage of all inflammatory affections of the respiratory tract.
- Bronchitis of young children.
- Short, painful, spasmodic cough, < morning and evening.
- Hemoptysis of pure blood; in pneumonia; after concussion or fall.
- Full, soft flowing pulse.

- Headache; throbbing; congestive; with earache; > nose bleed, cold application.
- Eyes red, inflamed with burning sensation.
- Violent earache. Acute otitis media.
- Hot cheeks with toothache.
- Vomiting; of bright red blood; of undigested food; ingesta; at irregular times.
- Stools; undigested; of bloody water; of yellow water. Dysentery.
- Hemorrhoids; inflamed or bleeding.

- Incontinence of urine from weakness of the sphincter. Diurnal enuresis.
- Menses; early; every three weeks; with heavy pain on vertex.
- Articular rheumatism; of shoulder; pain extend to chest and wrist, attack one joint after another, < slightest motion.
- Fevers; catarrhal, inflammatory, continued, infectious, pneumonia, intermittent, measles, hemorrhagic. Chill at 1 p.m.; with desire to stretch.

SURFACE MARKING OF KEYNOTES

GELSEMIUM SEMPERVIRENS

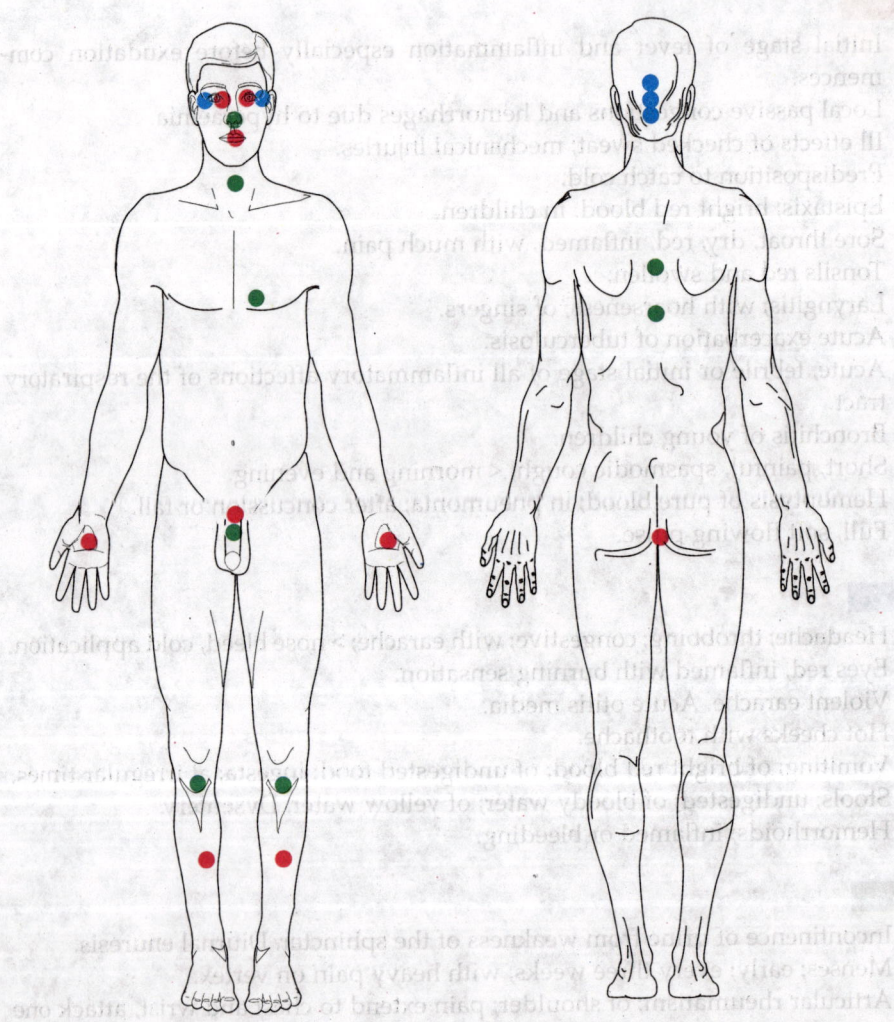

GELSEMIUM SEMPERVIRENS

Yellow Jasmine
Loganiaceae

- Dulness; dizziness, drowsiness; eye or visual effects; tremors; and polyuria accompany most of the ailments.
- Bad effects from fright, fear, exciting news and sudden emotions.
- The anticipation of any unusual ordeal, brings on diarrhea.
- Stage fright, nervous dread of appearing in public.
- Complete relaxation of the entire muscular system with motor paralysis.
- Lack of muscular co-ordination; confused; muscles refuse to obey the will.
- Weakness and trembling; of tongue, hands, legs; of the entire body.
- General depression from heat of sun or summer.

- Vertigo, spreading from the occiput; with diplopia, dim vision, loss of sight.
- Headache; preceded by blindness; beginning in the cervical spine; pain extending over the head; < by mental exertion, from smoking, heat of sun, lying with head low; > by profuse urination, shaking, lying with head high.
- Migraine begins at 2 or 3 a.m. > in the afternoon.
- Heavy drooping eyelids. Ptosis.
- Amaurosis from masturbation.

- Coryza, with thin acrid watery discharge.
- Paralytic dysphagia especially < from warm food.
- Incontinence from excitement; from paralysis of sphincter.
- Feeling as if heart would stop beating, if she did not move about.
- Weak slow pulse of old age.
- Knees weak < descending; tottering gait; cannot direct his legs.
- Chill without thirst, especially along the spine, running up and down the back; with aching and langour; mixed with heat or alternating with heat.
- Bilious remittent; malarial; typhoid; cerebro-spinal fevers.
- Measles.

SURFACE MARKING OF KEYNOTES

GRAPHITES

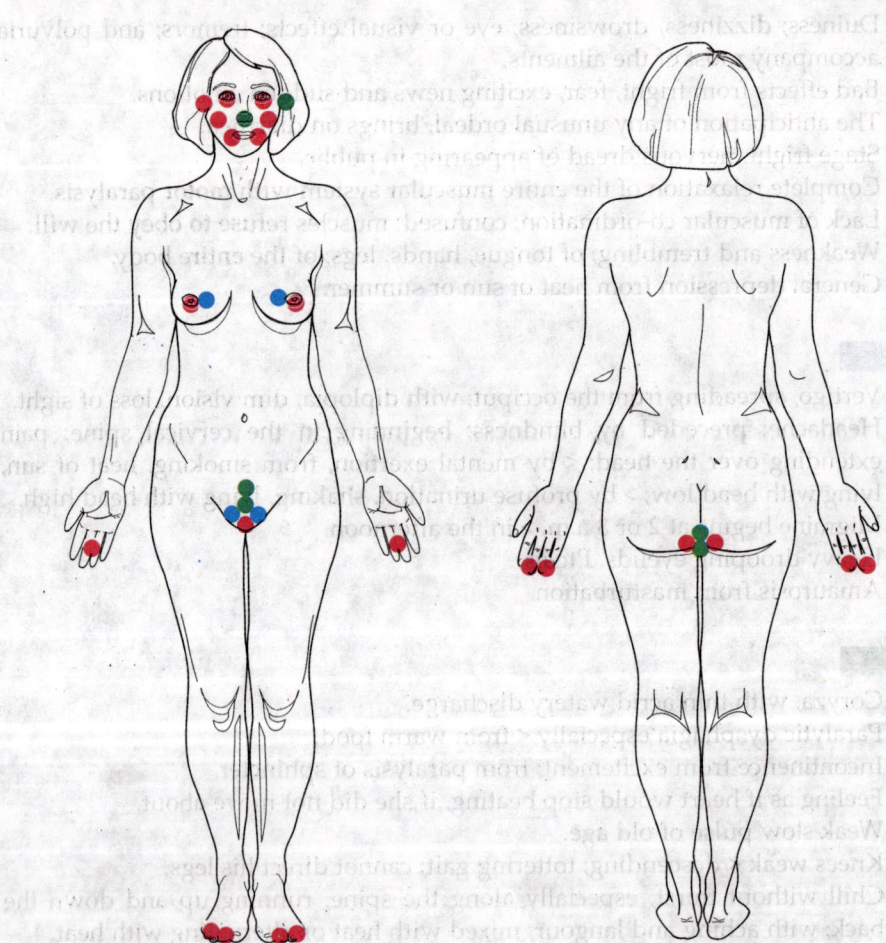

Skin ●●●●●
Mind ●●●●
Chilly ●

122 G

GRAPHITES

Black Lead
Amorphous Carbon

- Suited to women, inclined to obesity, relaxed, who suffer from habitual constipation and are chilly; a history of delayed menstruation.
- Unhealthy skin; every injury suppurates; old cicatrices break open again.
- Eruptions upon the ears, between fingers and toes on various parts of body, from which oozes a watery, transparent, sticky fluid.
- Eczema of lids; eruption moist and fissured; lids red and margins covered with scales or crusts.
- Cracks or fissures in ends of fingers, nipples, labial commissures; of anus; between the toes.
- Phlegmonous erysipelas: of face, with burning; stinging pain.
- The nails brittle, crumbling, deformed, thick and crippled; painful, sore, as if ulcerated.

- Sad, despondent; music makes her weep.
- Menses: too scanty, pale, late with violent colic; irregular; delayed from getting feet wet; with morning sickness and prostration.
- Leucorrhoea; acrid, excoriating; occurs in gushes day and night; before and after menses.
- Hard cicatrices remaining after mammary abscess, retarding the flow of milk.
- Cancer of breast, from old scars and repeated abscesses.

- Takes cold easily, sensitive to draft of air.
- Hears better in a noise.
- Diarrhea: stools brown, fluid, lienteric, offensive; after suppressed eruptions.
- Chronic constipation; stool difficult, too large, hard, knotty, stringy; followed by smarting sore pain in anus.
- Cataleptic condition; conscious, but without power to move or speak.
- Decided aversion to coition in both sexes.
- Sexual debility from sexual abuse.

SURFACE MARKING OF KEYNOTES

HELLEBORUS NIGER

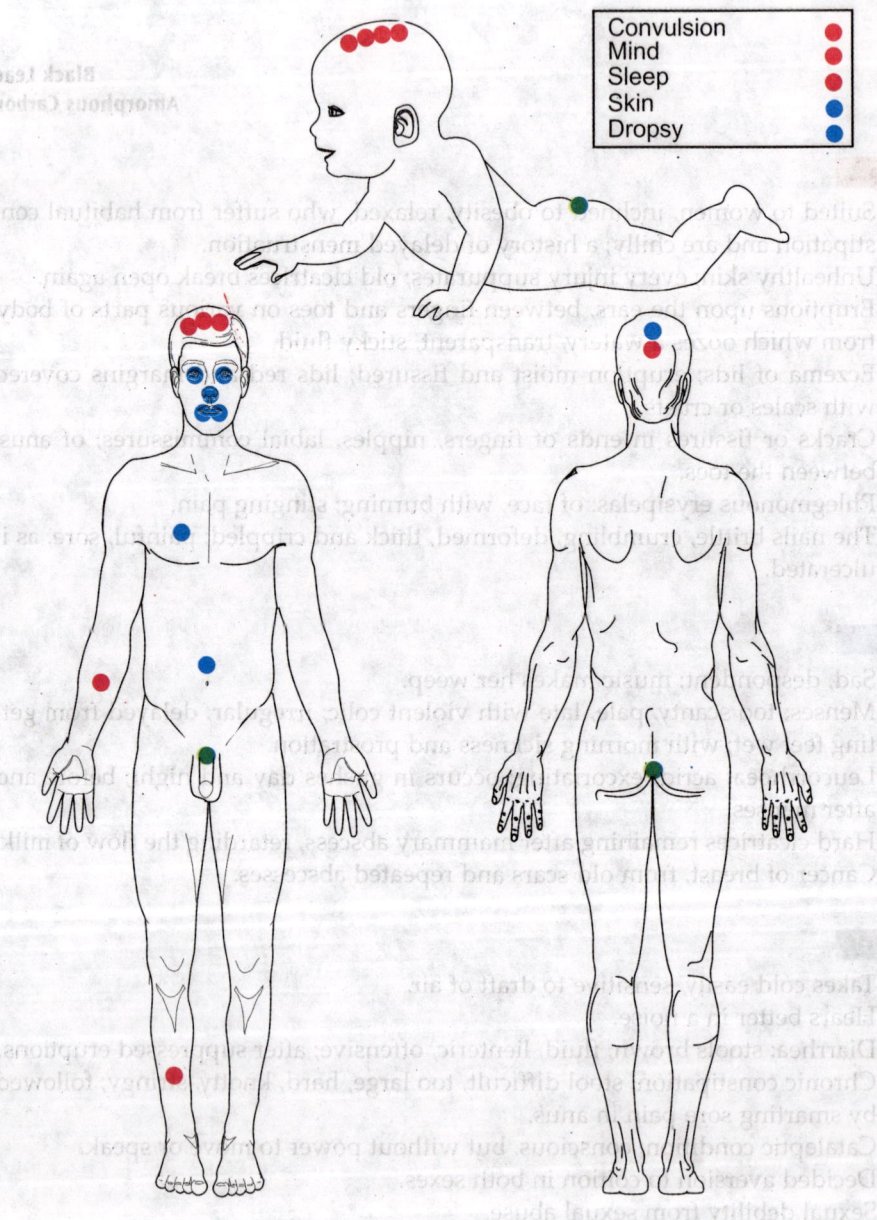

HELLEBORUS NIGER

Christmas Rose
Ranunculaceae

- Weakly, delicate, psoric children; prone to brain troubles; with serous effusion.
- Brain symptoms during dentition; threatening effusion.
- Meningitis: acute, cerebro-spinal, tubercular, with exudation; paralysis more or less complete; with the cri encephalique.
- Hydrocephalus post-scarlatinal or tubercular which develops rapidly.
- Boring head into pillow; rolling from side to side; beating head with hands.
- Convulsions with extreme coldness of body, except head or occiput which may be hot.
- Automatic motion of one arm and leg.
- Unconscious; stupid; answers slowly when questioned; a picture of acute idiocy.
- Greedily swallows cold water; bites spoon, but remains unconscious.
- Soporous sleep, with screams, shrieks, starts.

- Ill effects of checked exanthemata; blow, disappointed love.
- Dropsy: of brain, chest, abdomen; after scarlatina, intermittents; with fever, debility, suppressed urine; from suppressed exanthemata.
- Vacant, thoughtless staring; eyes wide open; insensible to light; pupil dilated, or alternately contracted and dilated.
- Constantly picking his lips, clothes, or boring into his nose with his fingers.
- Chewing motion of the mouth; corners of mouth sore, cracked; nostrils dirty and sooty, dry.

- Urine: red, black, scanty, coffee - ground sediment; suppressed in brain troubles and dropsy; albuminous. Uraemia.
- Diarrhea: during acute hydrocephalus, dentition, pregnancy; watery, clear, tenacious, colourless mucus; white, jelly-like mucus; like frog spawn; involuntary.

SURFACE MARKING OF KEYNOTES

HEPAR SULPHURIS

Christmas Rose
Ranunculaceae

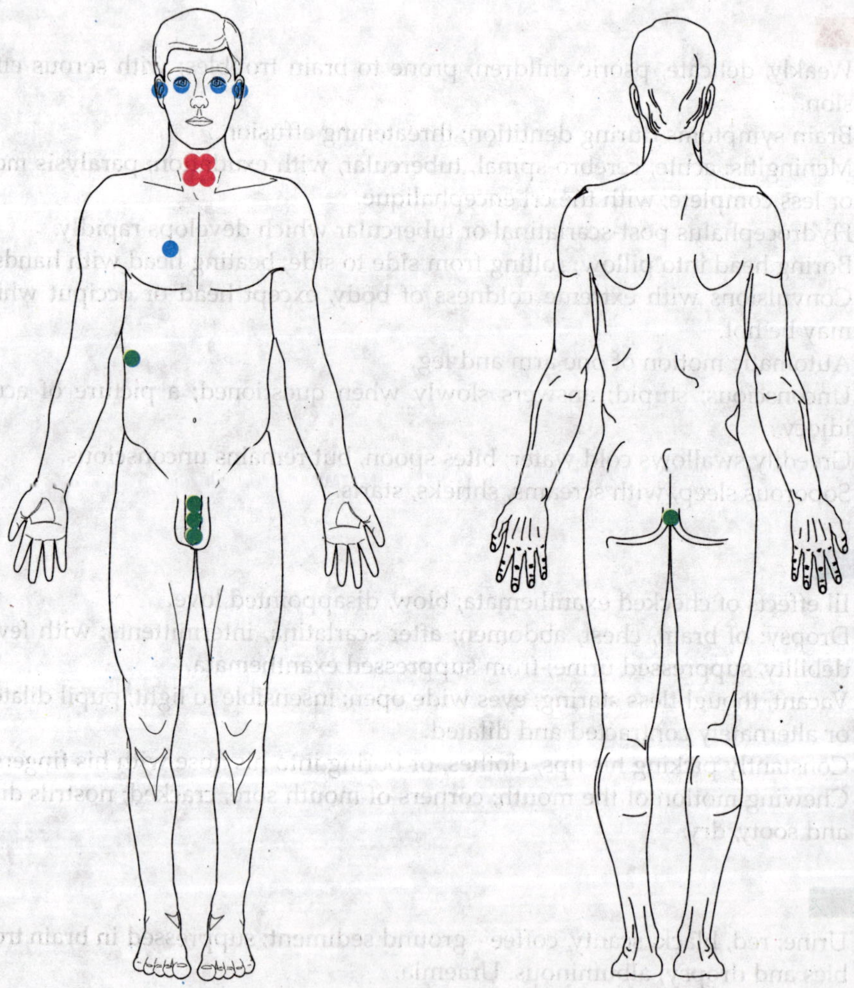

HEPAR SULPHURIS

Sulphurate of Lime
CaS

- Oversensitive, physically and mentally; the slightest cause irritates him.
- Extremely sensitive to cold air, imagines he can feel the air if a door is opened in the next room, must be wrapped up to the face even in hot weather.
- The skin is very sensitive to touch, cannot bear even clothes to touch affected parts, the pain often causing fainting.
- The slightest injury causes suppuration.
- Establishes suppuration around and removes foreign body.
- Cough: when any part of the body is uncovered; croupy, chocking, strangling from exposure to dry cold west wind, the land wind.
- Croup: deep, rough, barking cough, with hoarseness and rattling of mucus; expectoration loose, but cannot expectorate < cold air, cold drinks.
- Sensation of a splinter, fish bone or plug in the throat.
- Quinsy, when suppuration threatens; chronic hypertrophy, with hardness of hearing.

- Asthma; wheezing, rattling; short, deep breathing, threatens suffocation.
- Eyeballs: sore to touch. Ulcers on cornea.
- Fetid otorrhoea. Mastoiditis.
- Bad effects of suppressed exanthemata.
- Ulcers, herpes, surrounded by pimples or pustules and spread by coalescing.
- Sweats profusely day and night without relief but dare not uncover; sour, offensive; easily on slightest exertion.

- Diarrhea; stools sour, clay coloured; after drinking cold water.
- Hepatitis. Hepatic abscess.
- Urine: flow impeded, voided slowly, without force, drops vertically; must wait before it passes; some urine always remains in bladder.
- Flow of prostatic fluid after urination, during stool.
- Chancre like ulcers on prepuce.

SURFACE MARKING OF KEYNOTES

HYOSCYAMUS NIGER

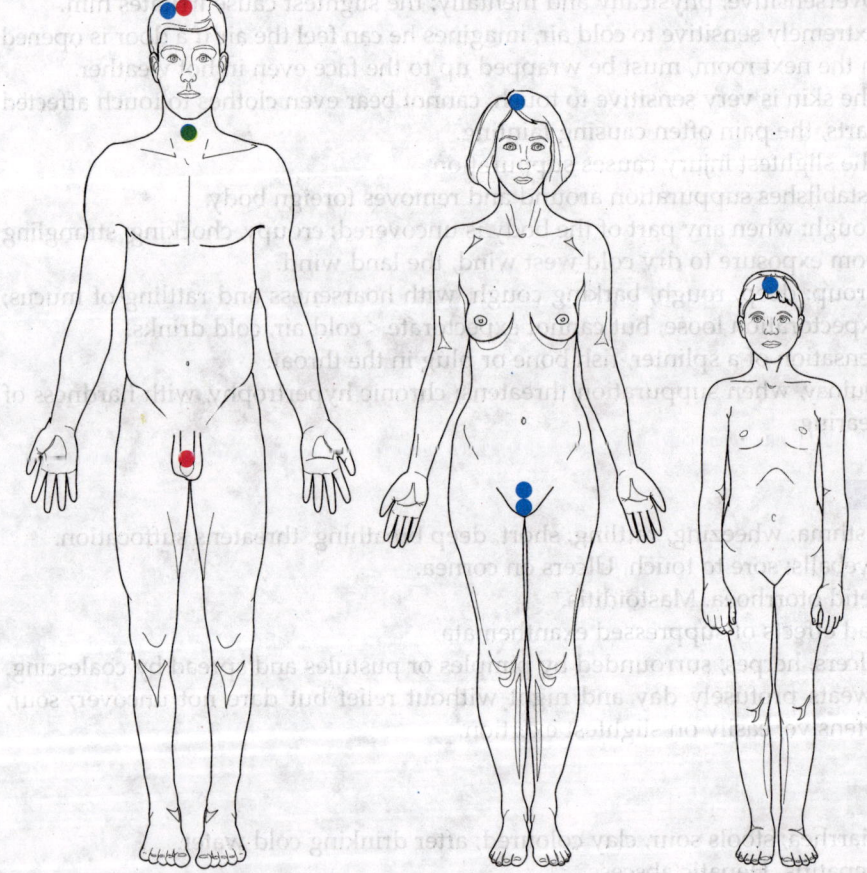

Mind	●●●●
Sleep	●●●
Spasms	●●
Fever	●

128 H

HYOSCYAMUS NIGER

Henbane
Solanaceae

- Diseases with increased cerebral activity, but non inflammatory in type; hysteria or delirium tremens; delirium, with restlessness.
- Fears: being alone; poison; being sold; to eat or drink; suspicious of some plot.
- Bad effects of unfortunate love; with jealousy, rage, incoherent speech or inclination to laugh at everything; often followed by epilepsy.
- Lascivious mania: immodesty, will not be covered, kicks off the clothes, exposes the genitals, plays with genitals; sings obscene songs.
- Intense sleeplessness of irritable, excitable persons from business embarrassments, often imaginary.

- Convulsions: of children, from fright or the irritation of intestinal worms; during labor, during the puerperal stage.
- Spasms: without consciousness, very restless; every muscle in the body twitches, from the eyes to the toes.
- Paralysis of bladder: after labor, with retention or incontinence of urine; no desire to urinate in lying in women.

- Cough; dry, nocturnal, hacking spasmodic; < lying, at night, after eating, drinking, talking, singing, > by sitting up.
- Fever: pneumonia, scarlatina, rapidly becomes typhoid; sensorium clouded, staring eyes, picking bed clothes, teeth covered with sordes, tongue dry and unwieldy; involuntary stool and urine; subsultus tendinum.

SURFACE MARKING OF KEYNOTES

IGNATIA AMARA

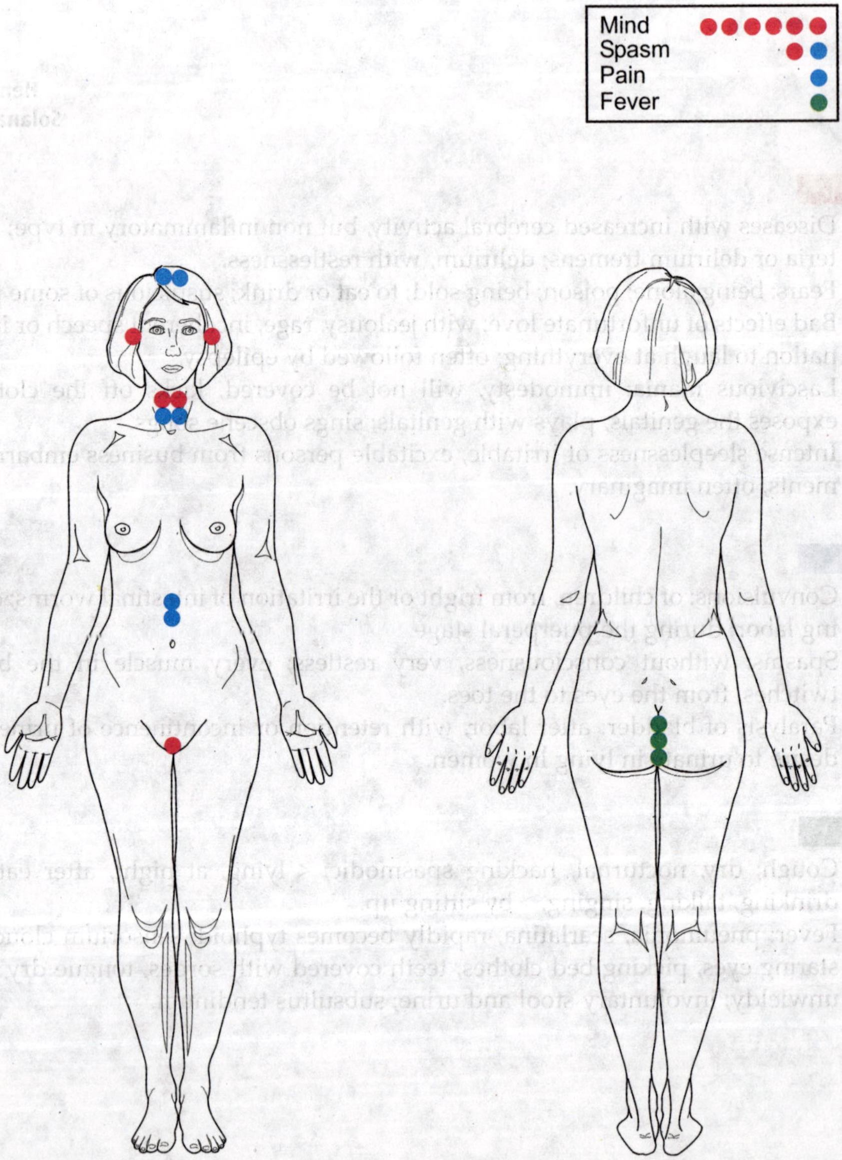

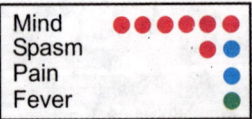

IGNATIA AMARA

St. Ignatius Bean
Loganiaceae

- Especially suited to nervous temperament; women of a sensitive, easily excited nature; dark hair and skin but mild disposition, quick to perceive, rapid in execution.
- Ill effects from suppressed mental sufferings, grief, fright, worry, anger, jealousy, disappointed love, old spinal injuries.
- Persons mentally and physically exhausted by long concentrated grief.
- Oversensitive and nervous. Highly emotional. Very moody. Easily offended.
- Changeable moods. Brooding grief. Silent and sad. Involuntary sighing.
- The remedy of great contradictions: the roaring in ears > by music; sore throat feels > when swallowing; cough < the more he coughs; cough on standing, still during a walk; spasmodic laughter from grief; sexual desire with impotency; the colour changes in the face when at rest.
- Twitchings, jerkings, even spasms of single limbs or whole body, when falling asleep.

- Cannot bear tobacco: smoking, or being in tobacco smoke, produces or aggravates headache.
- Headache, as if a nail was driven out through the side, > by lying on it.
- Pain in small circumscribed spots. Complaints return at precisely the same hour.
- Feeling as of lump, that can not be swallowed; > eating solids. Globus hystericus.
- Choking; spasms of glottis.
- Weak, empty feeling at pit of stomach; not > by eating; > by taking a deep breath.
- Hiccough: with eructations.
- Violent spasmodic yawning, with running from eyes.

- Plague; preventive and curative.
- Fever: red face during chill; thirst during chill only; > by external heat; heat without thirst, < by covering.
- Constipation; with excessive urging, felt more in upper abdomen; from carriage riding; of a paralytic origin; in habitual coffee drinkers.
- Prolapsus ani, < when the stool is loose; from straining, stooping or lifting.
- Hemorrhoids: prolapse with every stool, sharp stitches shoot up the rectum > when walking.

SURFACE MARKING OF KEYNOTES

IPECACUANHA

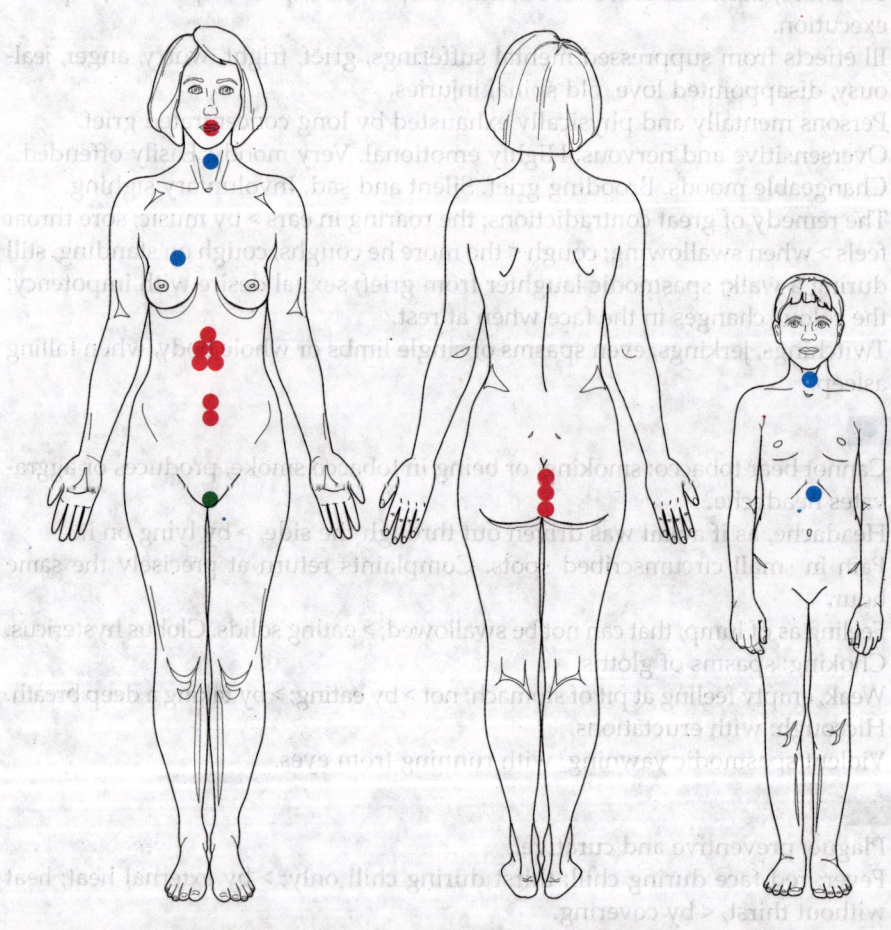

Pain	●
Haemorrhage	●
Fever	●

IPECACUANHA

Ipecac
Rubiaceae

- Adapted to cases where the gastric symptoms predominate; tongue clean or slightly coated.
- In all diseases with constant and continual nausea and shortness of breath.
- Nausea; with profuse saliva; vomiting of white, glairy mucus in large quantities, without relief; sleep afterwards; worse from stooping; the primary effects of tobacco; of pregnancy.
- Stomach: feels relaxed, as if hanging down.
- Clutching, squeezing, griping, as from a hand, each finger sharply pressing into intestines; worse from motion, > by repose.
- Flatulent, cutting colic about umbilicus. Cutting pains across abdomen from left to right.
- Intermittent dyspepsia, every other day at same hour; fever with persistent nausea.
- Stool: grassy - green; of white mucus; bloody; fermented, foamy, slimy like frothy molasses.
- Autumnal dysentery; cold nights, after hot days.
- Asiatic cholera, first symptoms, where nausea and vomiting predominate.

- Pains as if bones were all torn to pieces.
- Whooping-cough; child loses breath, turns pale, stiff and blue; strangling, with gagging and vomiting of mucus; bleeding from nose or mouth.
- Cough: dry spasmodic, constricted, asthmatic; with rattling of mucus in bronchi when inspiring; without expectoration, threatened suffocation from mucus.
- Violent dyspnoea. Gasps for breath.

- Hemorrhage: active or passive, bright red from all the orifices of the body.
- Uterine bleeding, profuse, bright, clotted, flow steady or gushing; with nausea and gasping; stitches from naval to uterus.
- Intermittent fever: with nausea in all stages; from gastric disturbance; heat without thirst; after suppression from quinine.

SURFACE MARKING OF KEYNOTES

KALI BICHROMICUM

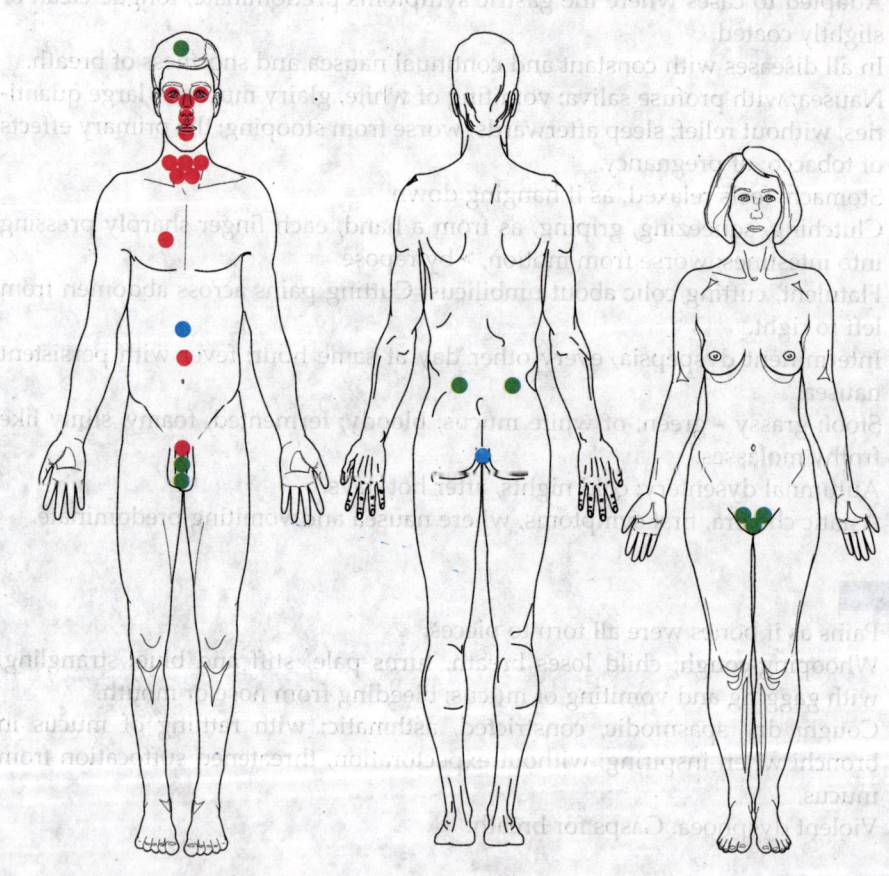

Pain •
Rheumatism •

134 K

KALI BICHROMICUM

Potassium Bichromate
$K_2Cr_2O_7$

🟥

- Affections of the mucous membranes eyes, nose, mouth, throat, bronchi; gastrointestinal and genitourinary tracts—discharge of a tough, stringy mucus which adheres to the parts and can be drawn into long strings.
- Nose: pressive pain in root of nose; discharge of plugs, "clinkers"; tough, ropy, green fluid mucus.
- Ulceration of septum, with bloody discharge or large flakes of hard mucus.
- Oedematous, bladder - like appearance of uvula.
- Diphtheria: prone to extend downwards to larynx and trachea.
- Deep-eating ulcers in fauces; often syphilitic.
- Croup: hoarse, metallic, with expectoration of tough mucus or fibro-elastic casts in morning on awakening with dyspnea > by lying down.

🟦

- Pains: in small spots; shift rapidly from one part to another; appear and disappear suddenly.
- Cracking of joints.
- Rheumatism alternating with gastric symptoms, rheumatism and dysentery alternate.
- Gastric complaints: loss of appetite; weight in pit of stomach; flatulence; < soon after eating; vomiting of ropy mucus and blood; round ulcer of stomach.

🟩

- Headache: blurred vision or blindness precedes the attack; must lie down; sight returns as headache increases.
- Prolapsus uteri, seemingly in hot weather.
- Leucorrhoea; acrid, yellow, ropy.
- Chancres ulcerating deeply.
- Sexual desire absent in fleshy people.
- Nephritis with scanty albuminous urine.
- Diseased conditions progress slowly but deeply; causing great weakness.

SURFACE MARKING OF KEYNOTES

KALI BROMATUM

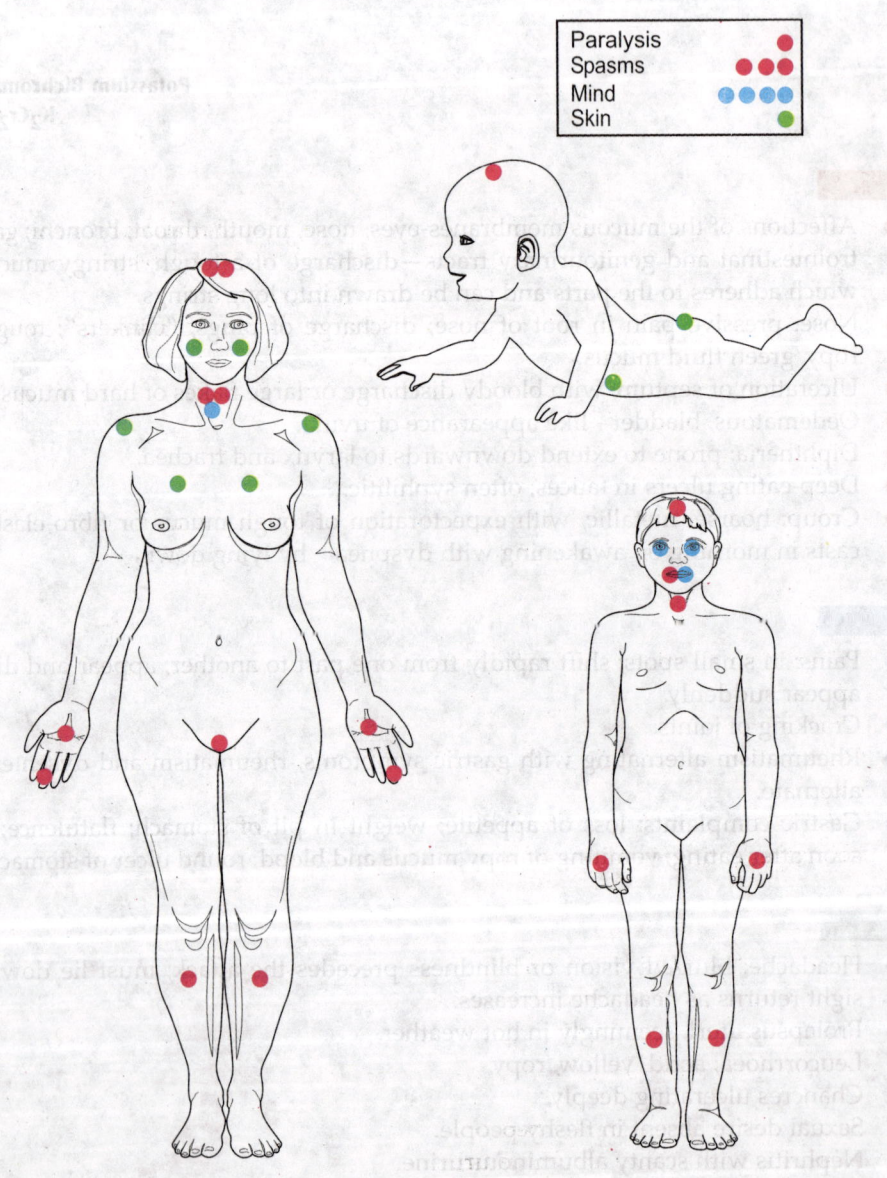

136 K

KALI BROMATUM

Potassium Bromide
KBr

- Adapted to large persons inclined to obesity; acts better in children than in adults.
- Inco-ordination of muscles; nervous weakness or paralysis of motion and numbness.
- Spasms: from fright, anger or emotional causes in nervous plethoric persons; during parturition, teething, whooping cough, bright's disease.
- Epilepsy: congenital, syphilitic, tubercular; usually a day or two before menses; at new moon; headache follows attack.
- Nervous, restless; cannot sit still, must move about or keep occupied.
- Hands and fingers in constant motion; fidgety hands; twitching of fingers.
- Staggering, uncertain gait; feels as if legs were all over sidewalk.
- Loss of sensibility, fauces, larynx, urethra, entire body.
- Stammering; slow, difficult speech.

- Loss of memory; forgets how to talk; absentminded; has to be told the word before he could speak it.
- Restlessness and sleeplessness due to worry, grief, loss of property or reputation, from business embarrassments, illness or death of a near friend, and sexual excess.
- Night terrors of children; grinding teeth in sleep, screams, moans, cries, followed by squinting. Somnambulism.
- Patient is sensual, with lascivious fancies; satyriasis and nymphomania.
- Nervous cough during pregnancy; dry, hard, almost incessant, threatening abortion.

- Onset of diseased condition is slow; without any pain.
- Cholera infantum, with reflex irritation of brain, before effusion.
- Daily colic in infants about 5 a.m.
- Acne: simplex, indurata, rosacea; bluish-red, pustular, on face, chest, shoulders; leaves unsightly scars.

SURFACE MARKING OF KEYNOTES

KALI CARBONICUM

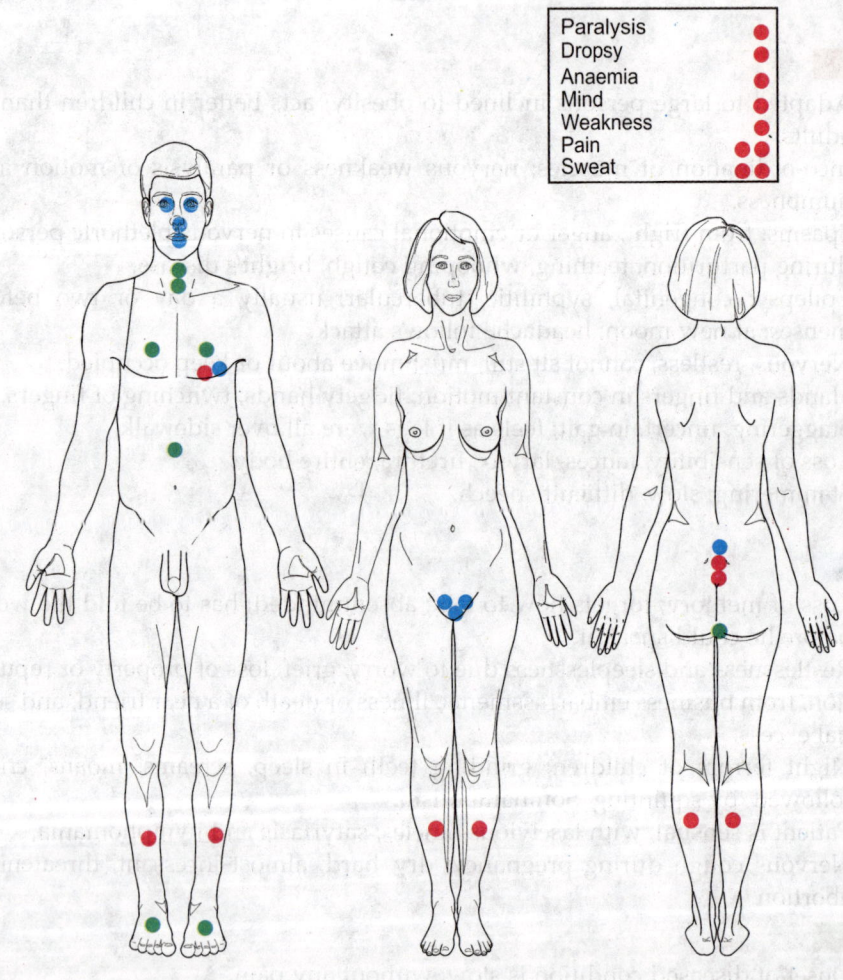

Paralysis
Dropsy
Anaemia
Mind
Weakness
Pain
Sweat

138 K

KALI CARBONICUM

Potassium Carbonate
$K_2 O_2 Co_2$

- For diseases of old people, dropsy and paralysis; with dark hair, lax fibre, inclined to obesity; soft, thin blooded, anemic and cold persons, always shivering.
- Great aversion to being alone.
- Weakness; of the muscles; of heart; of the back; of limbs; weakness of intellect.
- Pains stitching, darting, stabbing, worse during rest and lying on affected side.
- Backache, sweating, weakness; after abortion, labor, metrorrhagia; when eating; while walking feels as if she must give up and lie down; back feels as if broken.
- Legs give out; feel heavy. Soles very sensitive.
- Awakes at about 2 a.m. to 4 a.m. with nearly all complaints.
- Sweats; with slightest exertion; on painful part; on affected part.

- Nosebleed when washing the face in the morning.
- Bag-like swelling between the upper eyelids and eyebrows.
- Weak eyes; after coition, pollution, abortion, measles.
- Toothache only when eating; throbbing; < when touched by anything warm or cold.
- Heart; tendency to fatty degeneration; as if suspended by a thread.
- Pulse; small, soft, variable; intermittent or dicrotic.
- Feels badly, weak before menstruation; backache, before and during menses.
- Leucorrhoea; with labor like pains causing itching and burning in pudendum; > washing.
- Labor pains insufficient; violent backache; wants the back pressed.
- Menses; too late, scanty and pale discharge. Amenorrhoea.

- Cough: dry, spasmodic with gagging or vomiting of ingesta; hard, white masses fly from throat.
- Asthma; < from 2 to 4 a.m., least motion; > sitting up, bending forward or by rocking.
- Tubercular diathesis. Ulceration of the lungs.
- Difficult swallowing; with backache; food remains halfway in oesophagus.
- Stomach; distended, sensitive; excessive flatulency; feels as if it would burst.
- Constipation; stool large, difficult with stitching colic pains an hour or two before.
- Cannot bear to be touched; starts with a loud cry when touched ever so lightly, especially on the feet.

SURFACE MARKING OF KEYNOTES

KALI MURIATICUM

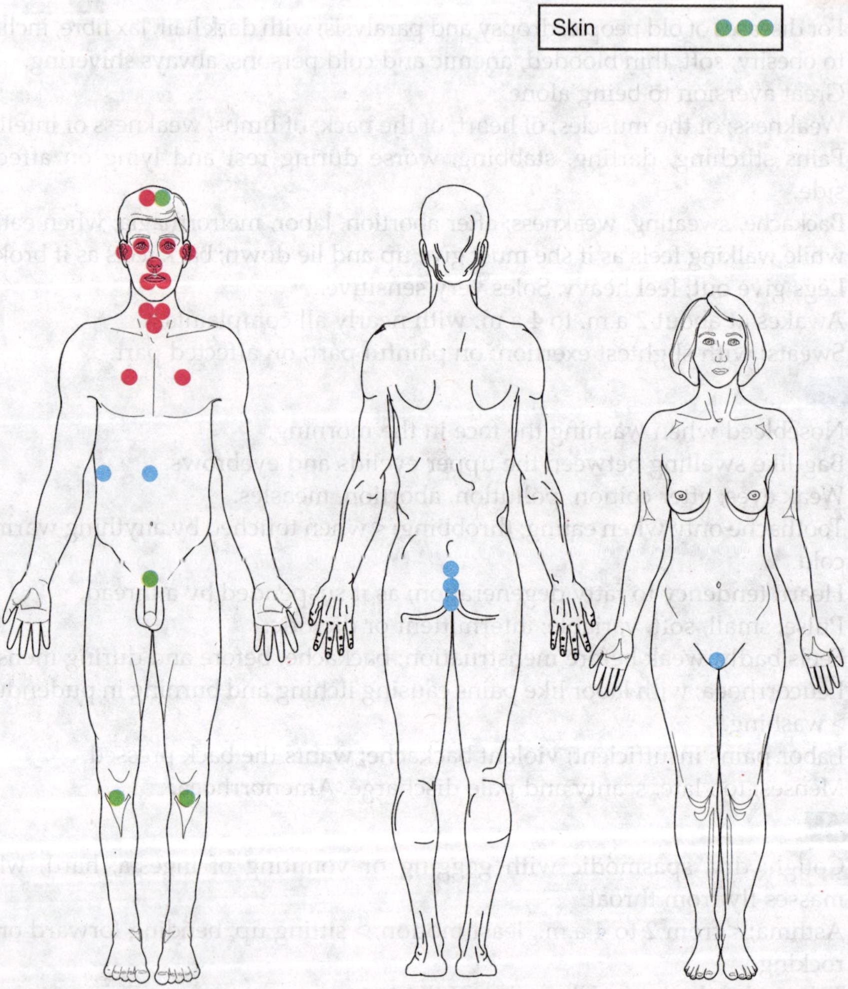

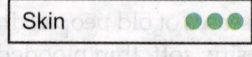

140 K

KALI MURIATICUM

Potassium Chloride
KCl

- Second stage of inflammations of serous membranes with tough, plastic or fibrinous exudates.
- It causes catarrhal condition, producing milky white, viscid, sticky, thick, slimy or lumpy discharges.
- Copious white dandruff.
- Cataract, corneal opacities.
- Deafness; from catarrhal condition and occlusion of Eustachian tubes.
- Crackling noises on blowing nose or swallowing.
- Aphthae, thrush, white ulcers in the mouth.
- Tongue; mapped; gray or white coating at the base.
- Grayish white, ulcerated, chronic sore throat; hawks out thick white mucus.
- Tonsils swollen; inflamed; swallowing excessively painful, can hardly breathe.
- Glandular swelling. Mumps without fever.
- Bronchitis; with thick white phlegm; difficult or oppressed breathing.

- Sore, cutting or sticking, shifting pains.
- Jaundice with sluggish action of liver.
- Fatty or rich food causes indigestion. Fulness after eating.
- Constipation; pale, hard or flocculent stools.
- Diarrhea in typhoid fever. Dysentery with shiny stools.
- Piles; bleeding, blood dark and thick.
- Leucorrhoea; milky white, thick, bland.

- Exudation and swelling around the joints.
- Ill effects of vaccination.
- Sprains. Burns. Blows. Embolism. Small pox. Measles. Chronic cystitis.
- Epilepsy after suppression of eruptions or eczema.
- Eruptions connected with stomach or menstrual disorders.

SURFACE MARKING OF KEYNOTES

KALI PHOSPHORICUM

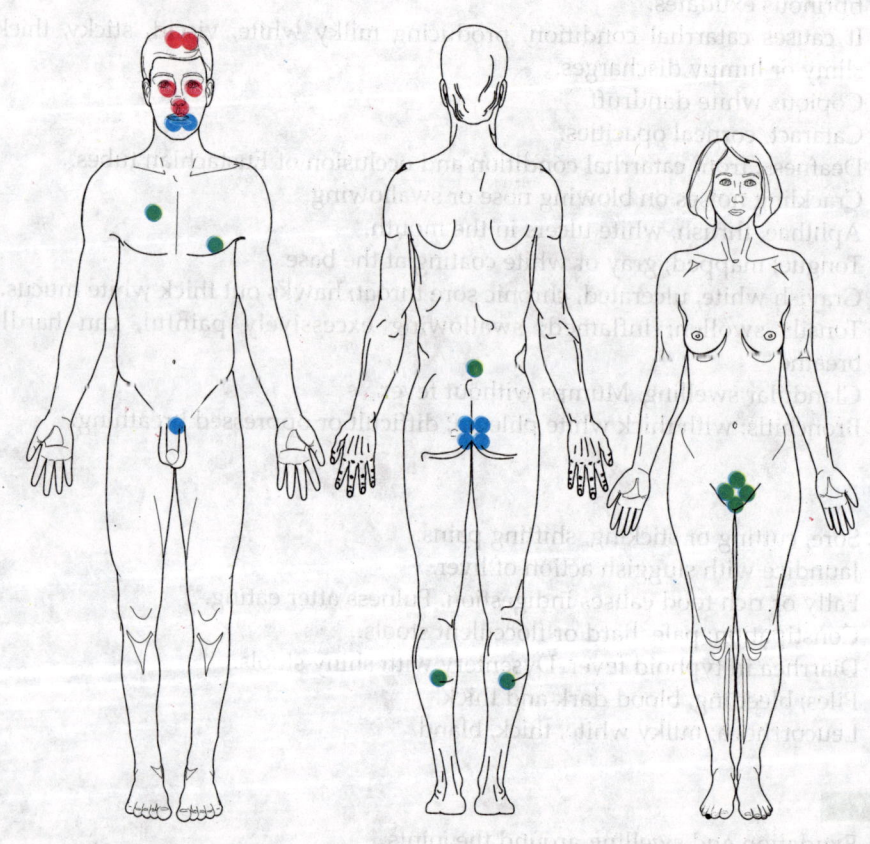

142 K

KALI PHOSPHORICUM

Potassium Phosphate
K$_2$HPO$_4$

- The patient is nervous, sensitive; weak and easily fagged; by slight causes like pain, worry, mental fatigue etc.
- Want of nerve power, neurasthenia.
- States of adynamia and decay; gangrenous conditions; suspected malignant tumors.
- Septic states and septic fevers.
- Paralytic weakness; or pain with paralytic sensation.
- Depression, anxiety, fear, despondency, irritability, restlessness, nervousness, suspicion, apprehension, night terrors, loss of memory, drowsiness, sleeplessness.
- Headache; of students; < before or during menses; > gentle motion, while eating.
- Cerebral anemia. Brain fag.
- Weakness of sight. Dropping of eyelids.
- Secretions; golden yellow; with putrid, carrion like odor.
- Hay fever. Violent sneezing. Itching in posterior nares.

- Mouth excessively dry. Speech slow, becoming inarticulate.
- Gums; spongy, receding, bleeding; with toothache.
- Diarrhea; painless, watery; foul, putrid odor, hot; golden yellow stools; from fright; with great prostration.
- Dysentery, stools consists of pure blood.
- Cholera, rice water stools.
- Flatulence; noisy, offensive.
- Nocturnal enuresis; in children and old people. Diabetes.

- Menses; irregular, too late, too scanty. Amenorrhoea.
- Periodical discharge of profuse orange colored fluid from vagina and rectum.
- Feeble and ineffectual labor pains. Favors parturition.
- Nervous asthma and palpitation, < going upstairs.
- Paralytic weakness of back and limbs.
- Subnormal temperature. Typhoid fever.

SURFACE MARKING OF KEYNOTES

KALI SULPHURICUM

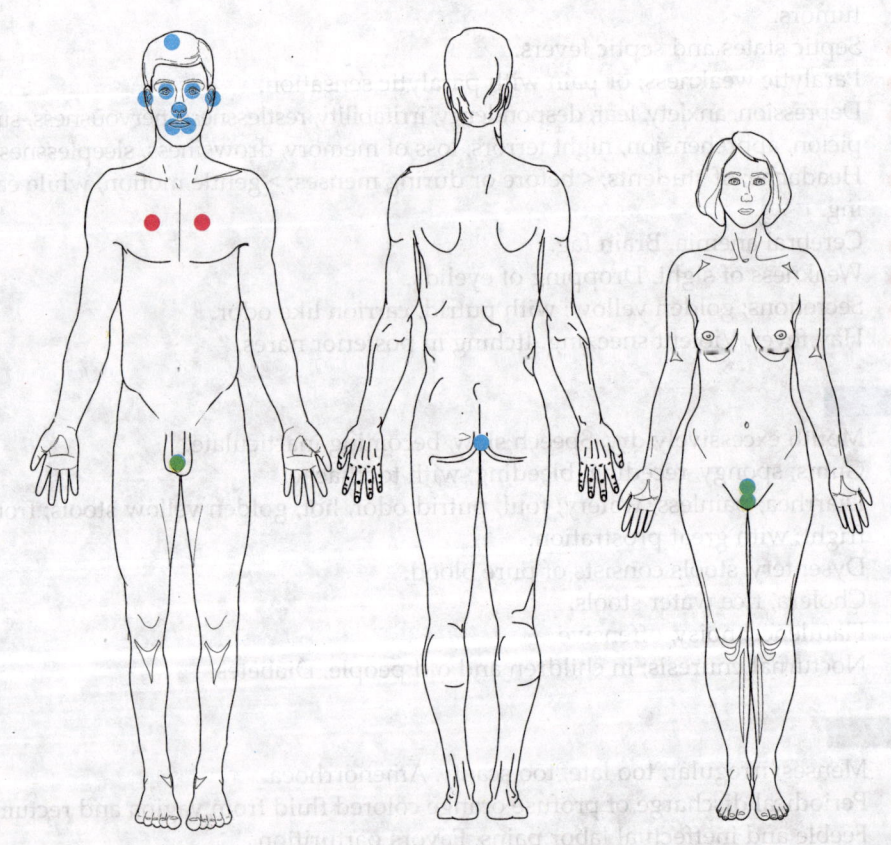

KALI SULPHURICUM

Potassium Sulphate
$K_2 SO_4$

- Affects respiratory mucous membranes and skin where it causes desquamation.
- Discharges are profuse, deep yellow, thin or sticky.
- Coarse rattling in chest with cough.
- Bronchial asthma; with easily expelled yellow, slimy expectoration.
- Ulcers, ooze thin yellow water.
- Psoriasis. Dry skin. Eczema. Measles.

- Stitching, tearing, shifting, wandering pains.
- Rheumatism worse by heat.
- Yellow dandruff; moist, sticky. Bald spots.
- Purulent yellow mucous in eye-diseases.
- Watery, sticky, thin, yellow, offensive discharge from ears.
- Engorgement of nasal mucosa with mouth breathing, after removal of adenoids.
- Yellow, slimy tongue.
- Yellow, slimy, watery, purulent diarrhea.

- Gonorrhea; gleet, slimy yellowish green discharge.
- Leucorrhoea; yellowish, watery.
- Intermittent fever; rise of temperature at night.
- Profuse, easy sweat.
- Suppurations. Third stage of inflammations.

SURFACE MARKING OF KEYNOTES

KREOSOTUM

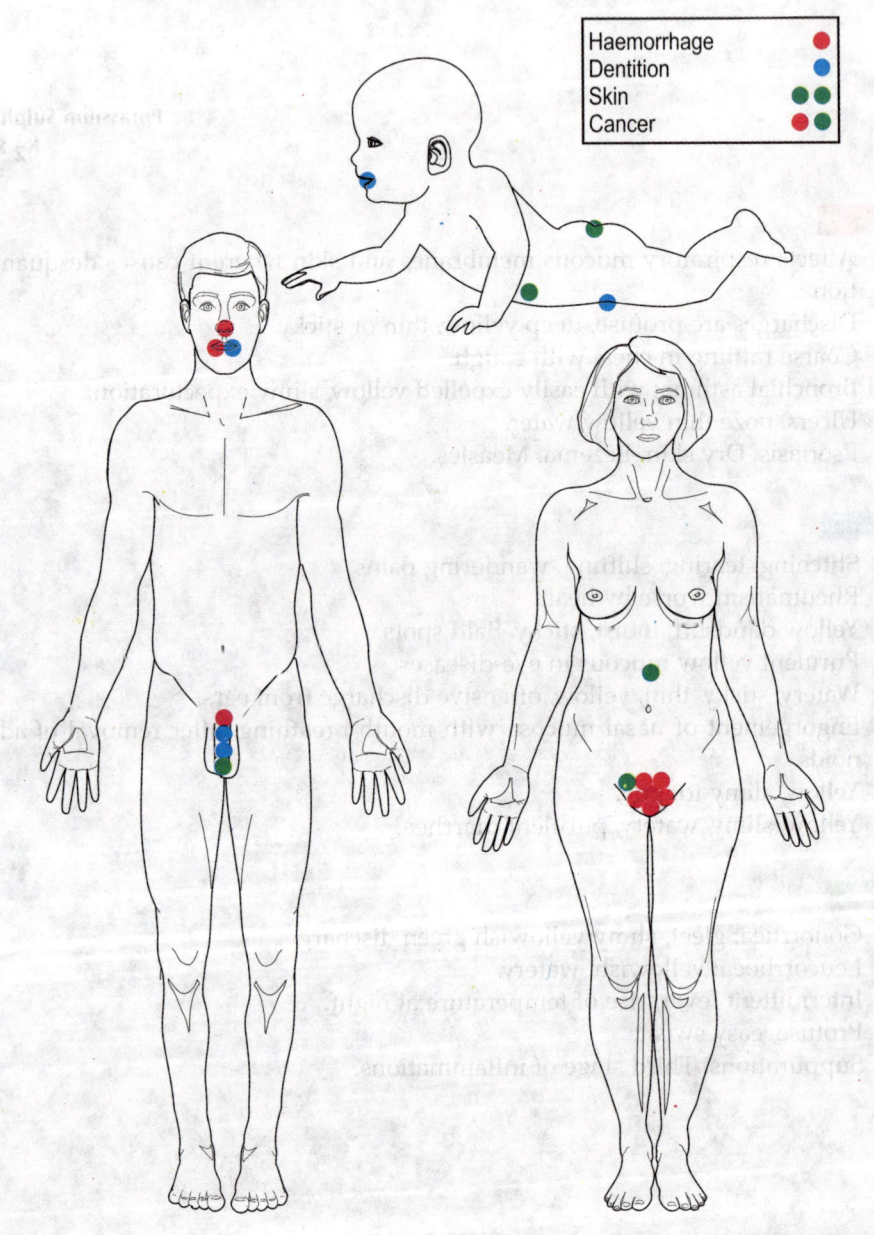

146 K

KREOSOTUM

Kreosote
A Distillation of Wood Tar

- It is suitable to lean persons, old women with post climacteric diseases; over grown, old looking; wrinkled, poorly developed, emaciated children.
- Hemorrhagic diathesis; small wounds bleed freely; flow passive, dark, oozing; in epistaxis, hemoptysis, hematuria, typhoid, tooth extraction.
- Profuse, corrosive, hot, fetid, ichorous discharges from mucous membranes.
- Menses: too early, profuse, protracted, intermittent; pain during, but < after it, > cold drinks; flow on lying down, cease on sitting or walking about.
- Before and during menses; headache; deafness.
- Leucorrhea; gushing; like blood water; offensive; corrosive; causing itching, staining the linen yellow; worse between periods; white; having odor of green corn.
- Cancer, erosion of cervix.
- Violent corrosive itching of pudenda and vagina.
- Lochia: dark, brown, lumpy, offensive, acrid; intermits.

- Painful dentition; teeth begin to decay as soon as they appear.
- Gums, bluish-red, soft, spongy, bleeding, inflamed, scorbutic, ulcerated with foetor oris.
- Enuresis; during first sleep, from which child is roused with difficulty.
- Incontinence of urine; can only urinate when lying; copious, pale, on coughing; urging, cannot get of bed quick enough.
- Smarting and burning during and after micturition.

- Vomiting; of pregnancy, sweetish water with ptyalism; of cholera, during painful dentition; incessant with cadaverous stool; in malignant affections of stomach.
- Itching, so violent toward evening as to drive one almost wild.
- Ulcers break out and heal; bleed after coition.
- Congenital syphilis. Cancerous affections. Gangrene.

SURFACE MARKING OF KEYNOTES

LACHESIS

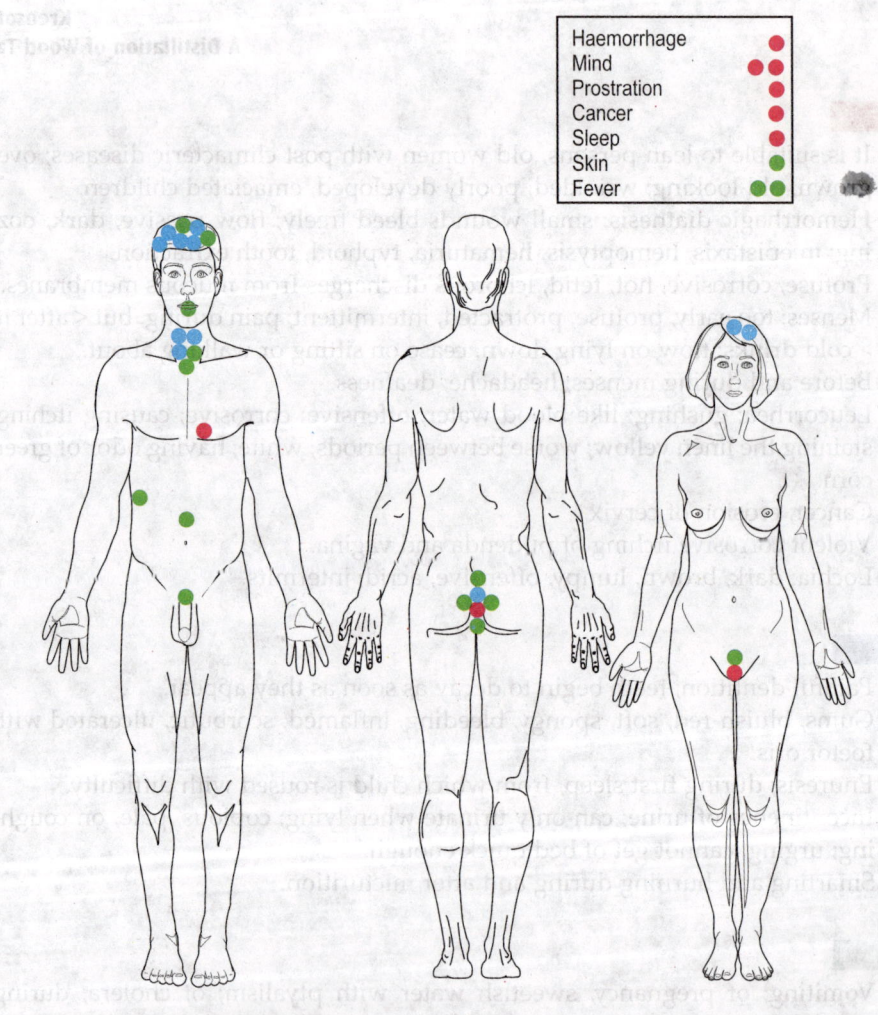

148 L

LACHESIS

Surukuku Snake Poison
Ophidia

- Better adapted to thin and emaciated than to fleshy persons; women of choleric temperament; climacteric ailments-piles, hemorrhages, palpitation, hot flushes and hot perspiration.
- Great loquacity, one word often leads into another story.
- Left side principally affected; diseases begin on the left and go to the right side.
- Great sensitiveness to touch; cannot bear bed-clothes or night-dress to touch throat or abdomen; clothes cause an uneasiness.
- Intensively rapid onset of the disease with great prostration.
- Malignant or septic states.
- All symptoms, especially the mental, worse after sleep, or sleeps into the aggravation; < in morning on waking.
- Hemorrhagic diathesis; small wounds bleed easily and profusely; blood dark, thin.
- Menses at regular time; too short, scanty, feeble, black; always better during menses.

- Drunkards with congestive headaches and hemorrhoids; prone to erysipelas or apoplexy.
- Suffocation and strangulation, on lying down; on dropping to sleep.
- Wants to be fanned, but slowly and at a distance.
- Diphtheria and tonsillitis, beginning on the left and extending to right side; dark purple appearance; < by hot drinks, after sleep; liquids more painful than solids when swallowing.
- Headache, < from motion, pressure, stooping, lying, after sleep.
- Rush of blood to head; after alcohol; mental emotions; suppressed or irregular menses; at climaxis; left-sided apoplexy.
- Epilepsy; comes on during sleep; from loss of vital fluids; onanism; jealousy.

- Sensation of constriction; in throat; on head; of anus; in rectum etc.
- Sensation of a lump in throat, abdomen, liver, rectum, bladder etc.
- Constipation: inactivity, stool lies in rectum, without urging.
- Piles: with scanty menses; at climaxis; strangulated.
- Boils, carbuncles, varicose ulcers with intense pain; malignant pustules; decubitus; dark, bluish, purple appearance; tend to malignancy.
- Fever: annually returning; paroxysm every spring; typhoid, typhus; stupor or muttering delirium.
- Tongue dry, black, trembles, is protruded with difficulty or catches on the teeth when protruding.
- Heat; on vertex; in flushes; on waking, on falling to sleep.

SURFACE MARKING OF KEYNOTES

LEDUM PALUSTRE

Rheumatism
Gout
Chilly
Pains
Arthritis
Injuries
Skin

150 L

LEDUM PALUSTRE

Marsh Tea
Ericaceae

- It is adapted to full-blooded, plethoric, robust or pale delicate patients with rheumatic, gouty diathesis; constitutions abused by alcohol.
- Complaints of people who are cold all the time; always feel cold and chilly; yet averse to external warmth.
- Parts cold to touch, but not cold subjectively to patient.
- Pains are sticking, tearing, throbbing; rheumatic pains are < by motion; < at night, by warmth of bed and bedcovering; > only when holding feet in ice water.
- Rheumatism or gout; begins in lower limbs and ascends; joints become the seat of nodosities and "gout stones," which are painful; acute and chronic arthritis.
- Affects left shoulder and right hip-joint.
- Swelling: of feet, up to knees; in heels as if bruised.
- Swelling of ankle with unbearable pain when walking, as from a sprain or false step.
- Ball of great toe swollen, painful.
- Easy spraining of ankle and feet.
- Back stiff; cramps in; < rising from sitting.

- If *Ledum* is given immediately after punctured wounds, it prevents tetanus.
- Punctured wounds by sharp-pointed instruments, as awls, nails; rat bites, stings of insects; the wounded parts especially are cold to touch.
- Long-remaining discolouration after injuries; "black and blue" places become green.
- Hemorrhage into anterior chamber after iridectomy.
- Contusions of eye and lids; ecchymosis of lids and conjunctiva.

- Much uric acid and sand in urine.
- Intense itching of feet and ankles, < from scratching, warmth of bed.
- Red pimples or tubercles on forehead and cheeks; as in brandy drinkers; stinging when touched.

SURFACE MARKING OF KEYNOTES

LYCOPODIUM CLAVATUM

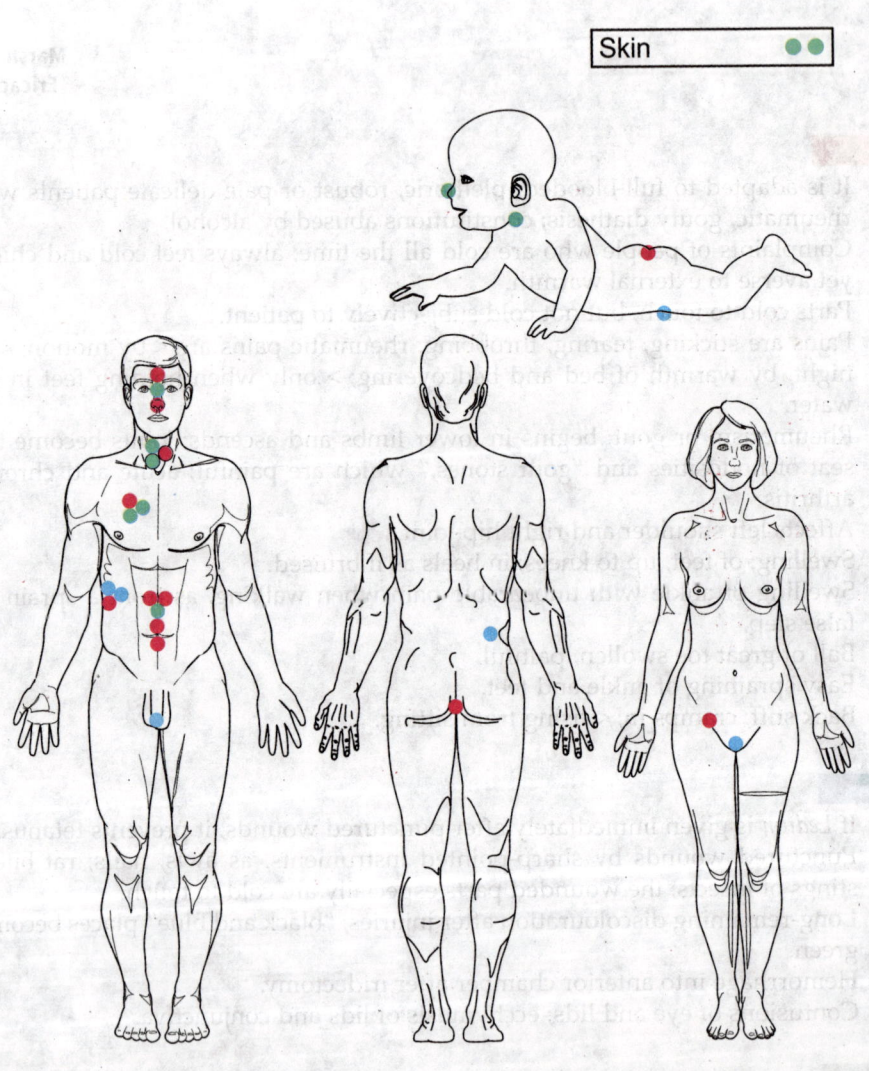

Skin

152 L

LYCOPODIUM CLAVATUM

Wolf's Foot; Club Moss
Lycopodiaceae

- For persons intellectually keen, but physically weak; upper part of body emaciated, lower part semi-dropsical; children and old people.
- Complexion pale, dirty, unhealthy; sallow, with deep furrows on forehead, look older than he is; fan like motion of alae nasi.
- Deep-seated, progressive, chronic diseases.
- Affects right side, or pain goes from right to left throat, chest, abdomen, liver, ovaries, < from four to eight p.m.
- Gastric affections: excessive accumulation of flatulence; loud, grumbling, croaking, especially in lower abdomen; fullness not relieved by belching.
- Good appetite but a few mouthfuls fill up to the throat and he feels bloated.
- Sour eructations, heart-burn, water brash, sour vomiting.
- Constipation: with ineffectual urging; since puberty; of infants; developing piles.

- Impotence: of young men, from onanism or sexual excess; old men, with strong desire but imperfect erections; falls asleep during coition, premature emission.
- Dryness of vagina; burning during and after coition.
- Red sand in urine, on child's diaper; child cries before urinating.
- Calculi; gall stones; renal colic right side.
- Chronic hepatitis; atrophic; nutmeg liver.

- Dry nose stopped at night, must breath through the mouth; snuffles, child starts from sleep rubbing the nose.
- Chronic catarrh; blows nose often.
- Diphtheria; fauces brownish-red deposit spreads from right tonsil to left, or descends from nose to right tonsils; < after sleep and from cold drinks.
- Cough; dry, tickling, teasing; day and night; in puny boys with emaciation.
- Pneumonia; neglected or maltreated, base of right lung involved especially.
- Brown spots on chest and abdomen.
- Periodically recurring boils. Chronic urticaria < warmth.

SURFACE MARKING OF KEYNOTES

MAGNESIA PHOSPHORICA

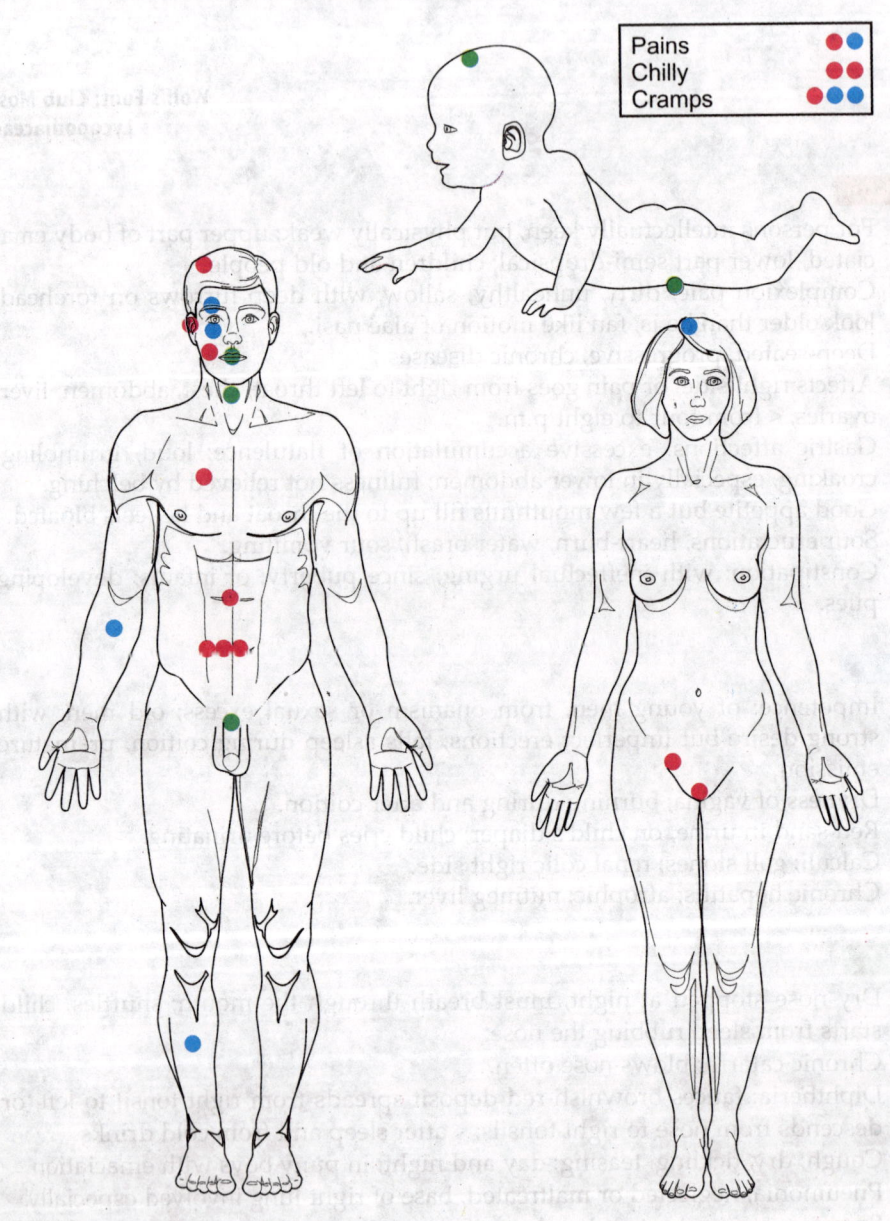

MAGNESIA PHOSPHORICA

Phosphate of Magnesia
$MgHPO_4 \cdot 7H_2O$

- Nervous, tense, and subject to sudden violent paroxysms of neuralgic pains; sharp, cutting, stabbing; shooting, stitching; lightning-like in coming and going; in periodic paroxysm; rapidly changing place; radiating, boring, constricting.
- Great dread of: cold air; uncovering; touching affected parts; moving.
- Complaints from: cold bathing or washing; standing in cold water; working in cold clay; catheterism; dentition; study.
- Affections of right side of body; head, ear, face, chest, ovary, sciatic nerve.
- Spasms or cramp of stomach, abdomen and pelvis, with clean tongue.
- Colic; flatulent, forcing patient to bend double; > by heat, rubbing and hard pressure.
- Menses: early; flow dark, stringy; pains < before, > when flow begins; > by heat and bending double; vaginismus; membranous dysmenorrhoea.

- Spasmodic effects; hiccough; yawning, chorea; twitchings; cramps etc.
- Cramps: of extremities; of writers, piano or violin players; during pregnancy.
- Headache: of school girls; from mental emotion, exertion or hard study; < 10 to 11 a.m. or 4 to 5 p.m.; > by pressure and external heat.
- Neuralgia: of face, supra or infra-orbital, ear; right side; intermittent; < by touch, cold air, pressure; > by external heat.

- Ailments of teething children; spasms during dentition, no fever.
- Toothache: at night; rapidly shifting; < eating, drinking, especially cold things; > by heat and hot liquids.
- Enuresis; nocturnal; from nervous irritation; after catheterization.
- Spasmodic, whooping cough > cool air.
- Always talking of her pains.
- Sleepy when attempting to study.

SURFACE MARKING OF KEYNOTES

MERCURIUS

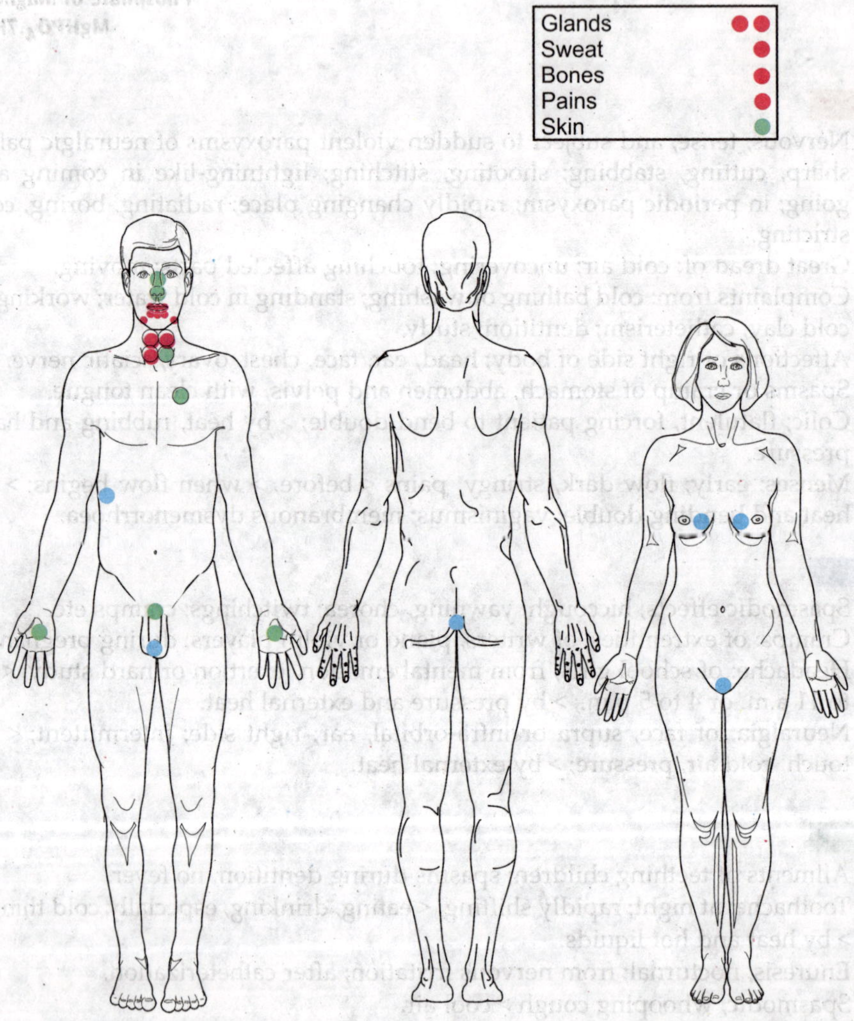

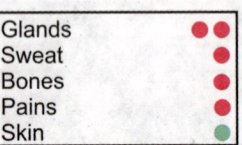

Glands	●●
Sweat	●●
Bones	●
Pains	●
Skin	●

156 M

MERCURIUS

Quicksilver
Hg

- Glandular swellings especially if suppuration be too profuse.
- Profuse perspiration attends nearly every complaint without relief.
- In bone diseases, pain worse at night.
- Ulcers on the gums, tongue, throat, inside of the cheek, with profuse salivation; irregular.
- Painful ragged, swollen, bleeding gums. Gumboil.
- Saliva: tenacious, soapy, stringy, profuse, fetid, coppery, metallic-tasting; flows during sleep.
- Tongue: large, flabby, shows imprint of teeth; red or white; mapped.
- Toothache: < in damp weather or evening air, warmth of bed, night, from cold or warm things; > from rubbing the cheek.
- Crowns of teeth decay, roots remain.
- Mumps, diphtheria, tonsillitis with profuse offensive saliva.
- Tonsils, inflamed, uvula swollen, elongated, constant desire to swallow.

- Liver; enlarged, sore; indurated. Jaundice.
- Dysentery: stool greenish, slimy, bloody, scanty, with colic and fainting; great tenesmus during and after, not > by stool, followed by chilliness and a "cannot finish" sensation.
- Glans and prepuce inflamed and swollen; phimoses.
- Leucorrhea: acrid, burning, itching with rawness; always worse at night; pruritus, < urinating, > washing with cold water.
- Mammae swelled, become hard with ulcerative pain during menses; milk in breasts instead of the menses.

- Catarrh: with much sneezing; fluent; acrid, corrosive; nostrils raw, ulcerated; yellow-green, fetid, pus-like, thick.
- Colds travel upwards or attack eyes.
- Cough; in double bouts; dry at night; yellow green sputum by day.
- Respiration difficult < lying on left side but cough < lying on right side.
- Frequent urging to urinate day and night, urinates more than drinks.
- Trembling extremities, especially hands, paralysis agitans.
- Cold swellings; abscesses, slow to suppurate.

SURFACE MARKING OF KEYNOTES

MERCURIUS CORROSIVUS

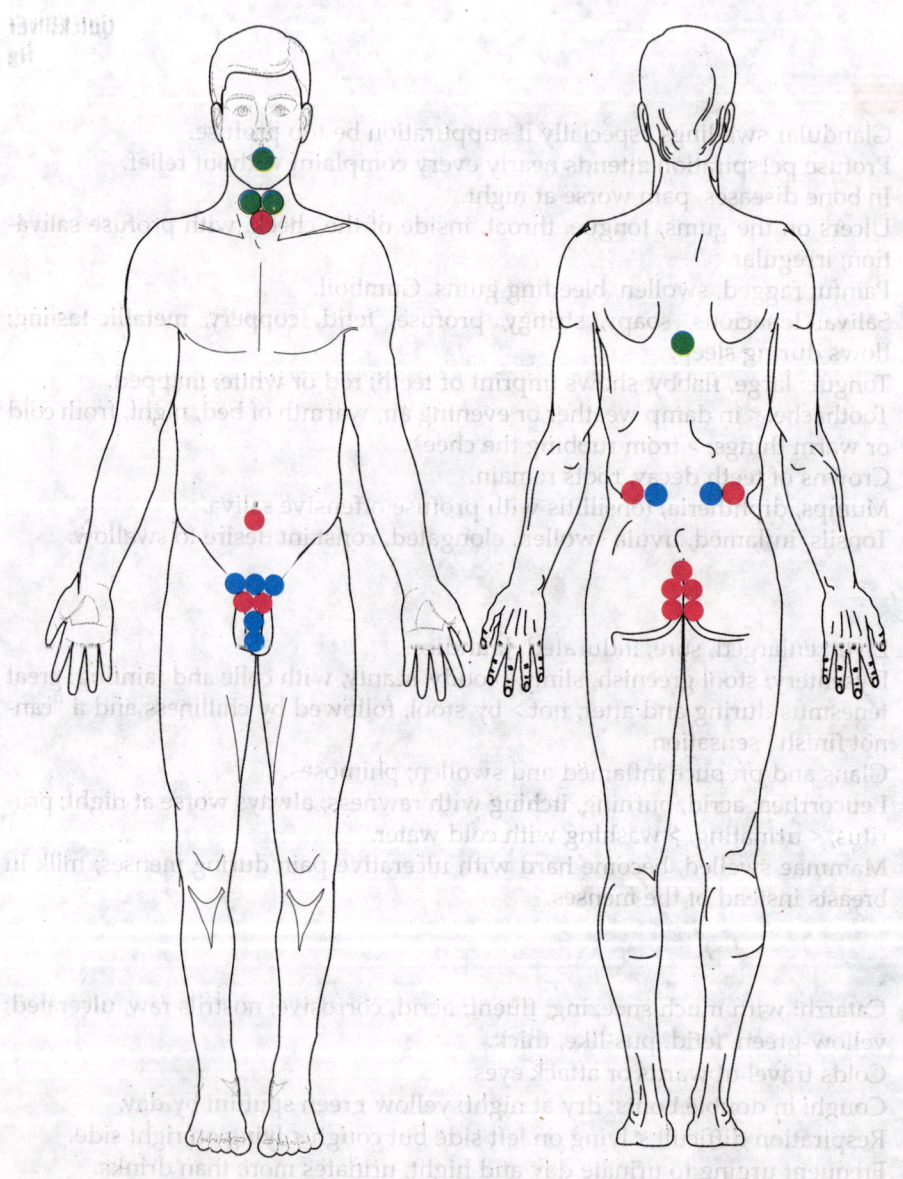

158 M

MERCURIUS CORROSIVUS

Corrosive Sublimate
HgCl$_2$

- Dysentery and summer complaints of intestinal canal, occuring from May to November.
- Inflammation with swelling, feeling of constriction and burning; in throat, rectum, neck of bladder, kidneys etc.
- Tenesmus: of rectum, not > by stool; incessant, persistent.
- Continuous urging to stool and urine; a never get done feeling.
- Stools; bloody, shreddy, scanty, offensive, slimy, hot with tormenting tenesmus.

- Tenesmus: of bladder, with intense burning in urethra.
- Urine hot, burning, scanty or suppressed; in drops with great pain; bloody, frequent.
- Albuminuria in early pregnancy.
- Bright's disease. Bleeding kidneys.
- Gonorrhea: second stage, thick greenish discharge, < at night; great burning and tenesmus.
- Syphilitic ulcers, with corroding, acrid pus.

- Gums; spongy; purple, swollen, with toothache.
- Burning pain and great swelling of throat < slightest pressure.
- Swallowing difficult; spasmodic constriction, on attempting to swallow a drop of liquid.
- Pott's disease, lies on back with knees drawn up.

SURFACE MARKING OF KEYNOTES

NATRUM CARBONICUM

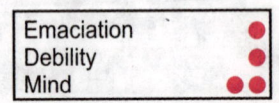

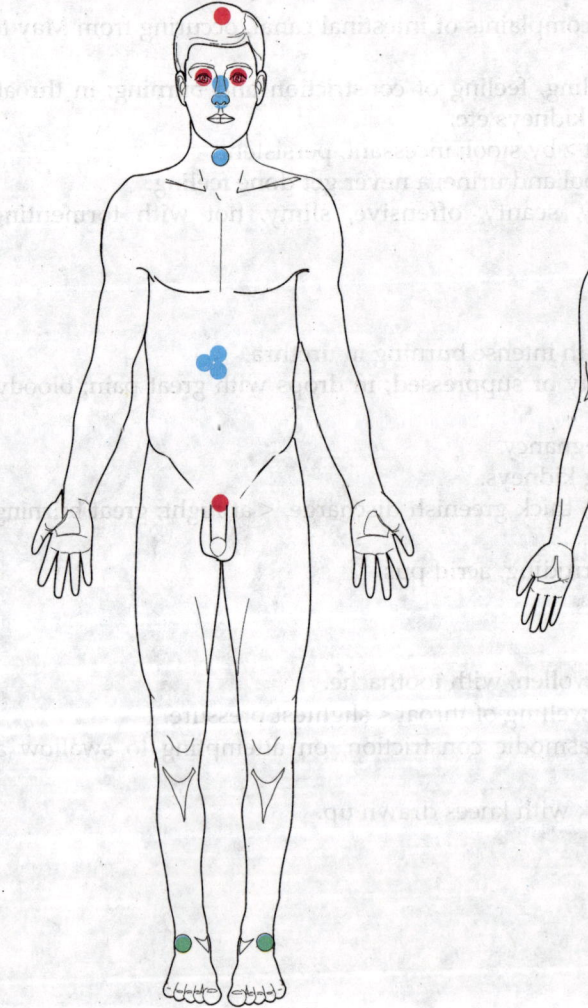

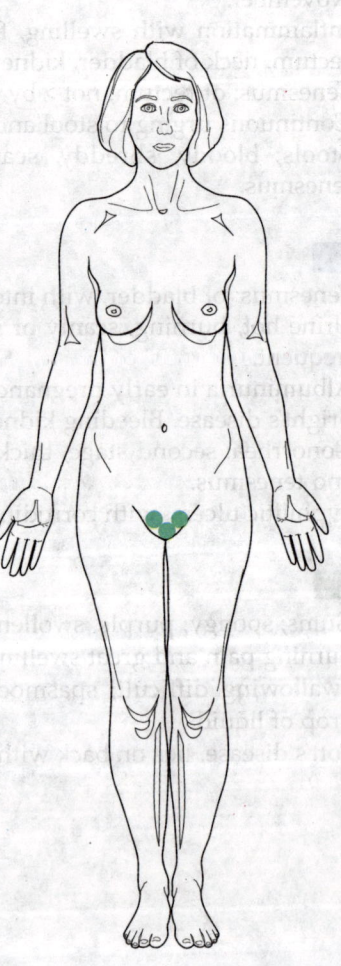

NATRUM CARBONICUM

Carbonate of Soda
$Na_2 Co_3 \; 10H_2O$

- Constitutions with aversion to open air and dislike to exercise, mental or physical.
- Emaciation with pale face and blue rings around the eyes, dilated pupils, dark urine; anemic; milky, watery skin and great debility.
- Great debility: caused by heat of summer exhaustion from least effort, mental or physical.
- Inability to thick or to perform any mental labor.
- Attacks of anxiety and restlessness during a thunder storm; < from music.
- Chronic effects of sunstroke.
- Headache: from slightest mental exertion; in hot weather; from sun or working under gaslight.

- Catarrh: extends to posterior nares and throat; hawking much thick mucus from throat.
- Profuse discharge during day, stopped at night.
- Thick, yellow, green, offensive, musty, hard discharge from nose; often ceasing after a meal.
- Digestion weak, < by slightest errors in diet.
- Aversion to milk; which causes diarrhea.
- Acid dyspepsia with belching and rheumatism, > by soda biscuits.

- Bearing down as if everything would come out; heaviness, < sitting, > by morning.
- Sterility from non-retention of semen.
- Discharge of mucus from vagina after an embrace, causing sterility. Promotes conception.
- Ankles weak; easy dislocation and spraining of ankle.

SURFACE MARKING OF KEYNOTES

NATRUM MURIATICUM

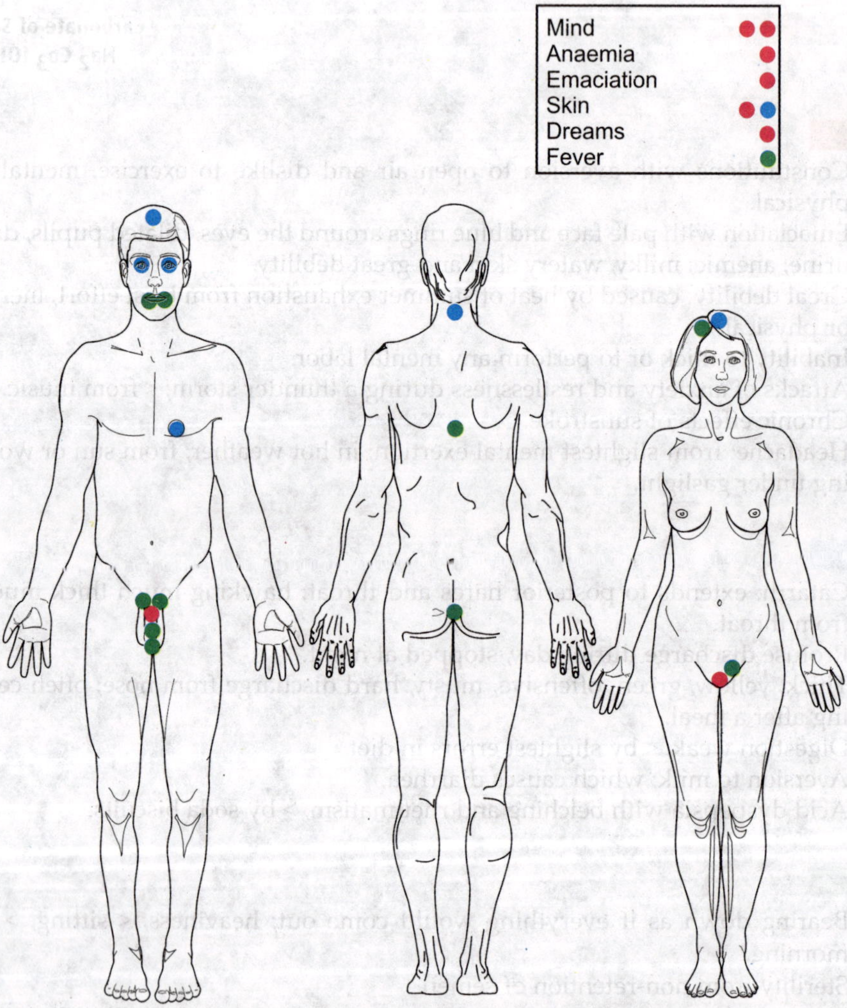

NATRUM MURIATICUM

Common Salt
NaCl

- Bad effects of anger, grief, fright, vexation, mortification or reserved displeasure.
- Sad weeping mood, without cause, but consolation from other < her troubles.
- Anemia or cachexia from loss of vital fluids, profuse menses, seminal losses, malaria.
- Great emaciation; losing flesh while living well.
- Bad effects of acid food, bread, quinine, excessive use of salts, cauterization with silver nitrate, from ocean voyage.
- Mucous membranes and skin may be dry or may produce thick, white or clear, watery, acrid discharges.
- Dreams: of robbers in the house; of burning thirst.

- Headache: bursting, maddening, hammering; over eyes; anemic, of school children; from eye strain; beginning with blindness; chronic; < on awakening, from sunrise to sunset, before, during and after menses, motion; > sleep, sweating.
- Lachrymation; from sneezing; coughing, laughing etc.
- Palpitation; shaking body; anxious, < exertion, emotion, lying on left side.
- Eczema; raw, red, inflamed, especially in edges of hair.
- Chaps of herpetic eruptions < flexures, or about knuckles.
- Urticaria, acute or chronic; over whole body, especially after violent exercise.

- Tongue: mapped, with red insular patches; like ring worm on sides.
- Heavy, difficult speech, children slow in learning to talk.
- Stools; dry, hard, crumbling; tears the anus or cause burning.
- Involuntary urination; on coughing; laughing; sneezing, walking, sitting.
- Has to wait long for urine to pass in the presence of others.
- Seminal emission soon after coition, with increased desire.
- Impotence, spinal irritation, paralysis, after sexual excesses.
- Intermittent fever: paroxysm at 10 or 11 a.m.; old, chronic, badly treated cases; chilly but < in sun.
- Prolapse of uterus with aching in lumbar region < in morning, > lying on back.
- Loss of hair in childbed or during lactation.

SURFACE MARKING OF KEYNOTES

NATRUM PHOSPHORICUM

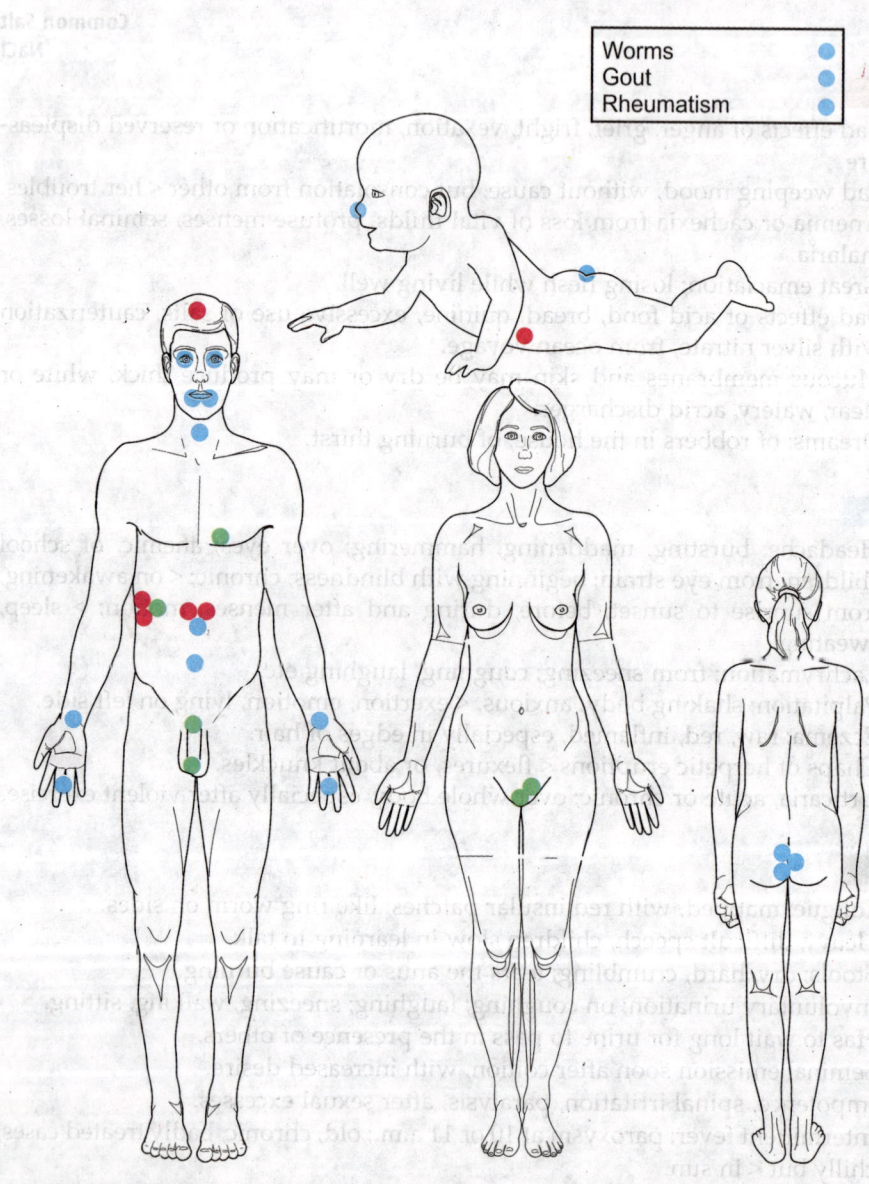

NATRUM PHOSPHORICUM

Sodium Phosphate
$Na_2HPO_4 \cdot 12H_2O$

- Conditions arising from excess of lactic acid, as a result of too much sugar.
- Infants who have been fed to excess, with milk and sugar.
- Ailments with excess of acidity.
- Cases of jaundice, hepatic colic, bilious headache, dyspepsia and imperfect assimilation of fats from lack of bile.
- Golden or deep yellow, creamy; discharges.

- Whites of the eyes dirty yellow.
- Yellow creamy coating at the base of tongue; on tonsils, or roof of mouth.
- Sour eructations, sour vomiting, greenish diarrhea.
- Intestinal, round or thread worms, with symptoms of acidity, itching and picking of the nose, grinding of teeth, occasional squinting, colic, itching at the anus, restless sleep etc.
- Gout and acute inflammatory or articular rheumatism.
- Aching in wrists and finger joints.

- Urging to stool and urination after coitus in men.
- Emissions followed by weak back and trembling of knees.
- Sterility; with acid secretions from vagina.
- Leucorrhoea; sour, creamy, honey colored or acid or watery.
- Sclerosis of liver and hepatic form of diabetes.
- Heart pains alternating with rheumatic pains.

SURFACE MARKING OF KEYNOTES

NATRUM SULPHURICUM

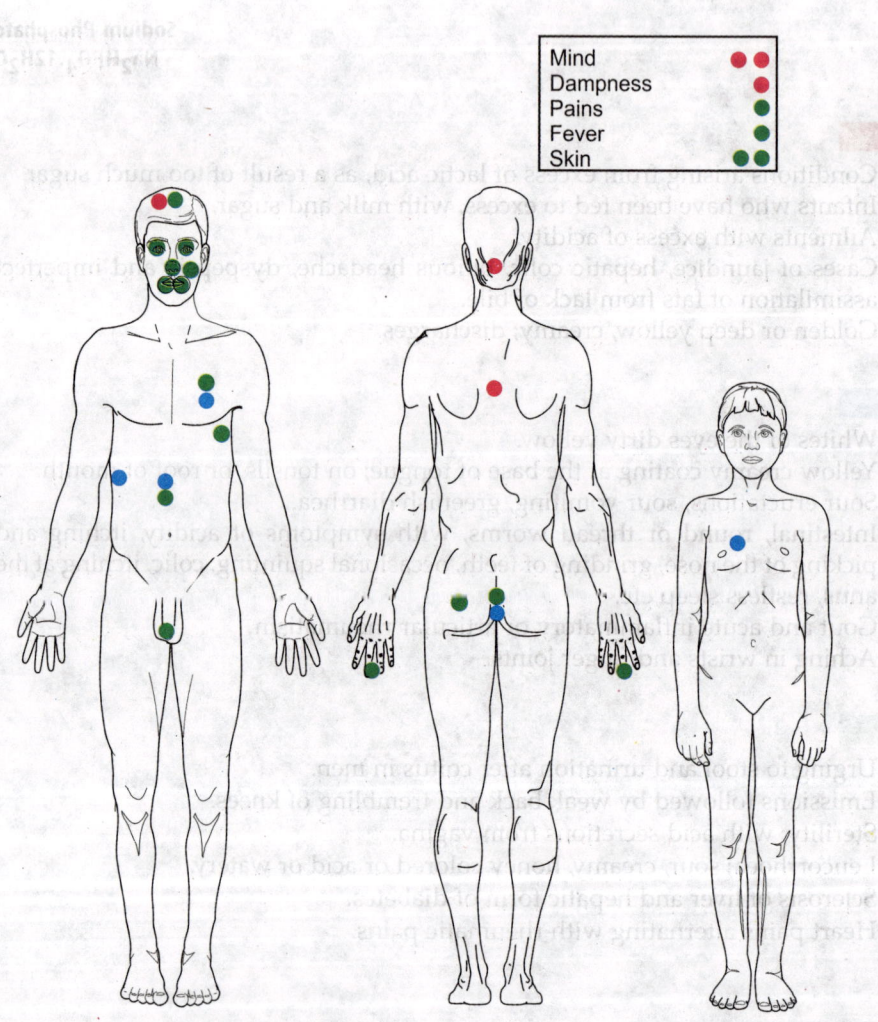

Mind
Dampness
Pains
Fever
Skin

NATRUM SULPHURICUM

Sodium Sulphate, Glauber's Salt
$Na_2SO_4 \cdot 10H_2O$

- Mental effects from injuries to head; chronic brain effects of blows, falls.
- Ailments which are < by, or which depend upon, dampness of weather, damp houses or cellars, patient feels every change from dry to wet.
- Recovers slowly from every sickness.
- Depressed; lively music makes her sad; satiety of life.
- Spinal meningitis: violent crushing gnawing pains at base of brain; head drawn back; spasms with mental irritability and delirium.

- Humid asthma in children; with every change to wet weather; with every fresh cold; always worse in damp, rainy weather; < early morning; sputa greenish, copious. Constant desire to take deep, long breath.
- Sycotic pneumonia: lower lobe of left lung; great soreness of chest, during cough, has to sit up in bed and hold the chest with both hands.
- Acid dyspepsia with heart burn and flatulence. Green bilious vomiting.
- Liver region sore, tender; < deep breathing; stepping; jar; heavy, < lying on left side.
- Diarrhea: bilious; rumbling, gurgling in bowels, followed by sudden noisy spluttering stools, much flatus; on first rising and standing on the feet; or drives from bed; after a spell of wet weather.

- Granular lids like small blisters; green pus and terrible photophobia < morning.
- Nose bleed before and during menses, stops and returns often.
- Dirty brown, or greenish yellow, thick, pasty tongue especially at base.
- Toothache > by cold water, cool air.
- Diabetes mellitus caused by a lessened secretion of pancreatic fluid.
- Gonorrhea: greenish-yellow, painless, thick discharge; chronic or suppressed.
- Piercing pains; at short ribs (left); in hip (left) < rising or sitting down.
- Inflammation around root of nails.
- Intermittent and bilious fevers.
- Vesicles, eruptions containing yellow, watery secretions.
- Tendency to warts around eyes, scalp, face, chest, anus etc.

SURFACE MARKING OF KEYNOTES

NITRIC ACID

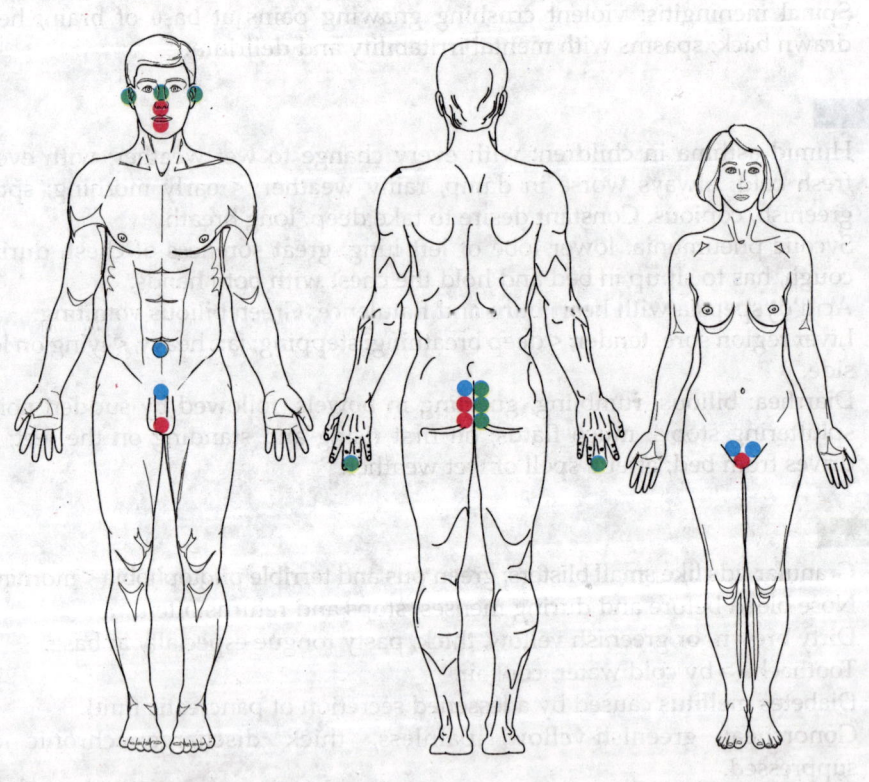

NITRIC ACID

Acidum Nitricum
HNO$_3$

- Especially suited to thin persons of rigid fiber, dark complexion black hair, and eyes, of spare habit; or persons suffering from chronic diseases, having a tendency to catch cold or diarrhea.
- Irritable, head strong; hateful and vindictive; inveterate, illwilled, unmoved by apologies.
- Anxiety about his disease, fear of cholera; of death.
- Sensation: of a band; of a splinter in affected parts.
- Affects especially the muco-cutaneous junction of the body; mouth, nose, rectum, anus, urethra, vagina.
- Pains: sticking, pricking as from splinters; suddenly appearing and disappearing; ulcerative gnawing.
- Discharges are acrid, thin, offensive, dirty yellowish green or brown; causes redness or destroy hair.

- Hemorrhage: bright, profuse or dark; from over exertion of body; from bowels in typhoid; from rectum after removal of piles; after miscarriage or postpartum; after curettage.
- Ulcers rapid, raw, easily bleeding, zig-zag, ragged, with proud flesh or plugs of pus.
- Warts, condylomata: large, jagged, pedunculated; bleeding readily on washing or touch; moist, oozing.
- Caries and exostoses of bones.
- Urine: scanty, dark brown, strong-smelling, "like horse's urine"; cold when it passes; turbid.

- Pain as if rectum or anus were torn or fissured.
- Violent cutting pains in anus even after soft stool, lasting for hours.
- Painful, easily bleeding piles.
- Deafness; > noise, in trains, riding in carriage; after measles.
- Ozena: green casts from the nose every morning.
- Nails, distorted, discolored, yellow, curved, ingrowing.

SURFACE MARKING OF KEYNOTES

NUX MOSCHATA

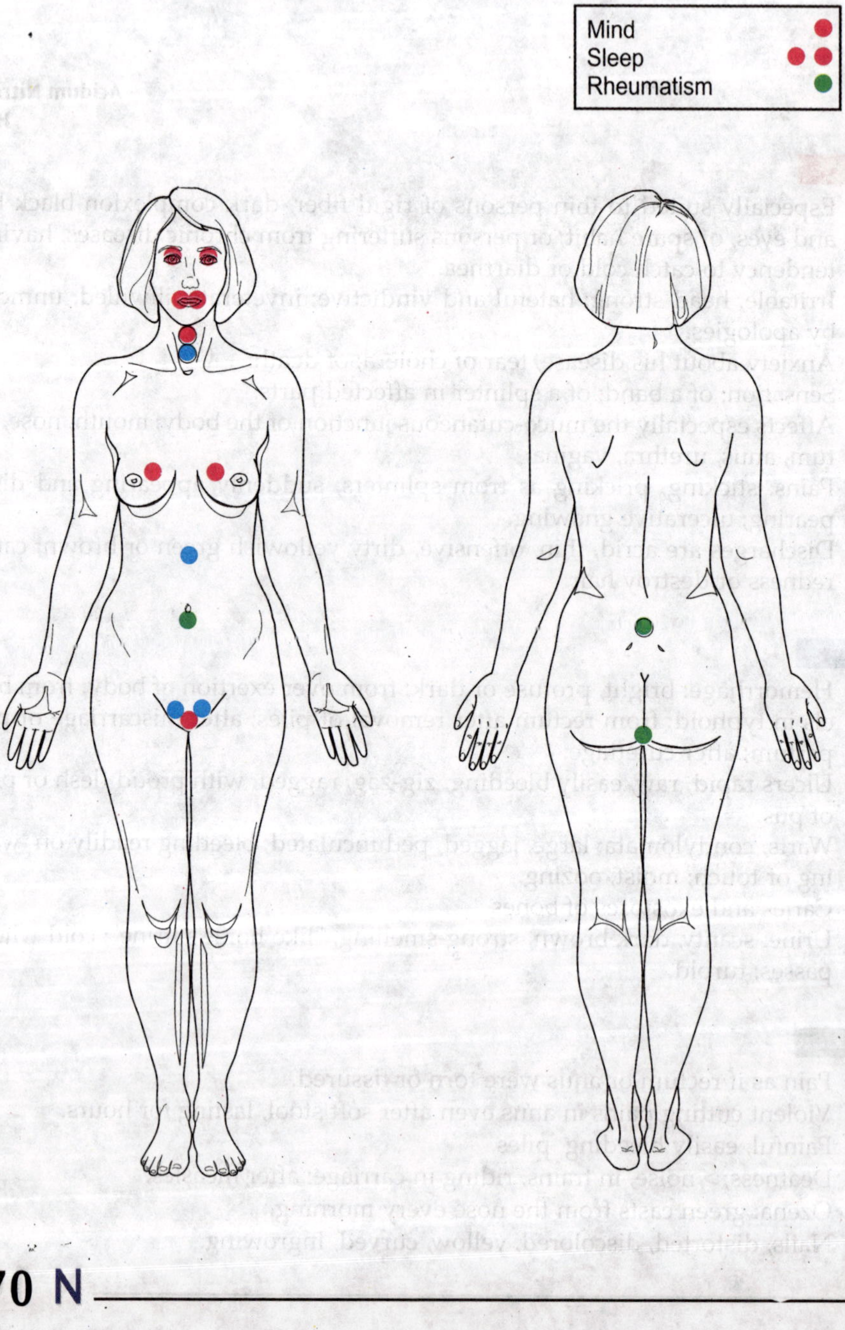

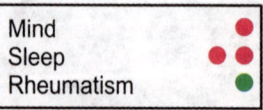

170 N

NUX MOSCHATA

Nutmeg
Myristicaceae

- It is useful to scrawny, delicate, hysterical women who have small breast and who laugh or cry by turns; complaints of pregnancy to people with a dry skin, who rarely perspire.
- Thoughts suddenly vanish, while talking, reading or writing.
- Marked tendency to fainting fits; < at stools, at menses, with slight pain.
- Great sleepiness with all complaints.
- Stupor and insensibility; unconquerable sleep.
- Great dryness of the mouth; tongue so dry it adheres to roof of mouth; throat dry, stiffened, no thirst.
- Dryness of eyes; too dry to close the lids.

- Menses; irregular, in time and quantity; thick dark.
- Leucorrhoea; muddy, bloody; in place of menses.
- Pain, nausea and vomiting during pregnancy; from wearing pessaries.
- Sudden hoarseness, < from walking against the wind.

- Abdomen enormously distended after every meal.
- Diarrhea: in summer, from cold drinks; epidemic in autumn, white stools; from boiled milk; during dentition; during pregnancy.
- Rheumatic affections: from getting feet wet; from exposure to drafts of air while heated; < in cold, wet weather, or cold wet clothes; > warmth.
- Backache, while riding in carriage.

SURFACE MARKING OF KEYNOTES

NUX VOMICA

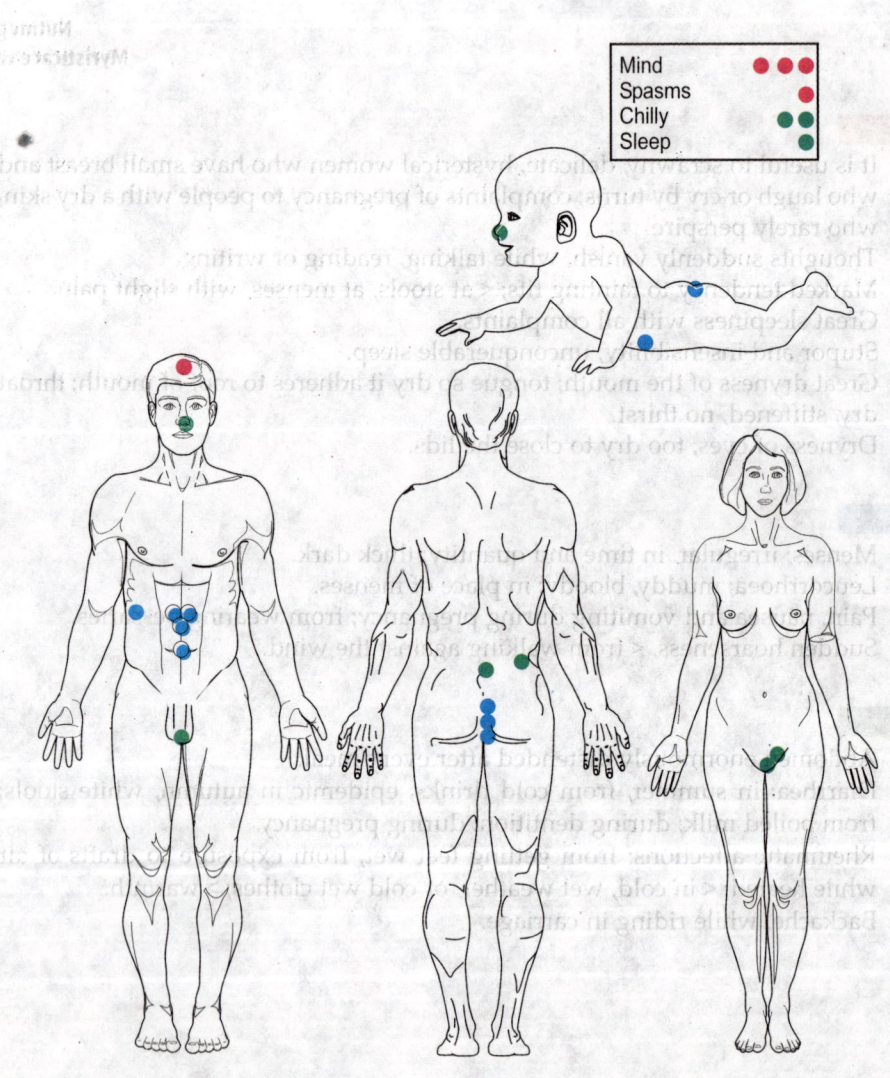

Mind	● ● ●
Spasms	● ●
Chilly	● ● ●
Sleep	● ●

NUX VOMICA

Poison Nut
Loganiaceae

- Adapted to thin, spare, careful, zealous, active subjects with dark complexion, hypochondriac, literary, studious persons, drunkards who lead a sedentary life and disposed to be irritable, quarrelsome, spiteful, malicious, nervous and melancholic.
- Violent, excitable, angry, impatient, head-strong, self-willed.
- Oversensitive to external impressions; to noise, odors, touch, light or music; trifling ailments are unbearable.
- Bad effects of: coffee, tobacco, beer, alcoholic stimulants; drugs, highly spiced or fat food; over eating, sedentary habits, high living, night watch.
- Tendency to faint: from odors; in morning; after eating; after every labor pain.
- Convulsions, tetanic, with consciousness; < anger, emotion, touch, moving > by grasping tightly.

- Nausea: constant; after eating; in morning; from smoking; > if he can only vomit.
- Eructations; difficult; sour, bitter.
- Food lies like a heavy knot in stomach.
- Jaundice; from anger.
- Constipation; with frequent unsuccessful desire, passing small quantities of feces; sensation as if not finished.
- Alternate constipation and diarrhea.
- Piles itching, blind, bleeding, > cool bathing.
- Hernia; infantile; from constipation or crying; umbilical; strangulated.

- Snuffles of infants.
- Coryza, dry at night, fluent by day and open air.
- Body burning hot especially face, but unable to move or uncover without feeling chilly.
- Easily chilled, must be covered in every stage of fever-chill, heat or sweat.
- Renal colic (right), extending to genitals and legs; with dribbling urine.
- Bad effects of onanism; sexual excess.
- Lumbago, must sit up to turn over in bed.
- Menses; profuse, early and prolonged; intermittent; irregular; with fainting spells.
- Labor pains: Violent, spasmodic; cause urging to stool or to urinate.
- Sleepy in the evening while sitting or reading hours before bedtime, and awakes at 3 or 4 a.m., falls into a dreamy sleep at daybreak but on waking feels wretched.

SURFACE MARKING OF KEYNOTES

OPIUM

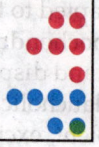

Low vitality
Sleep
Weakness
Mind
Paralysis

174 O

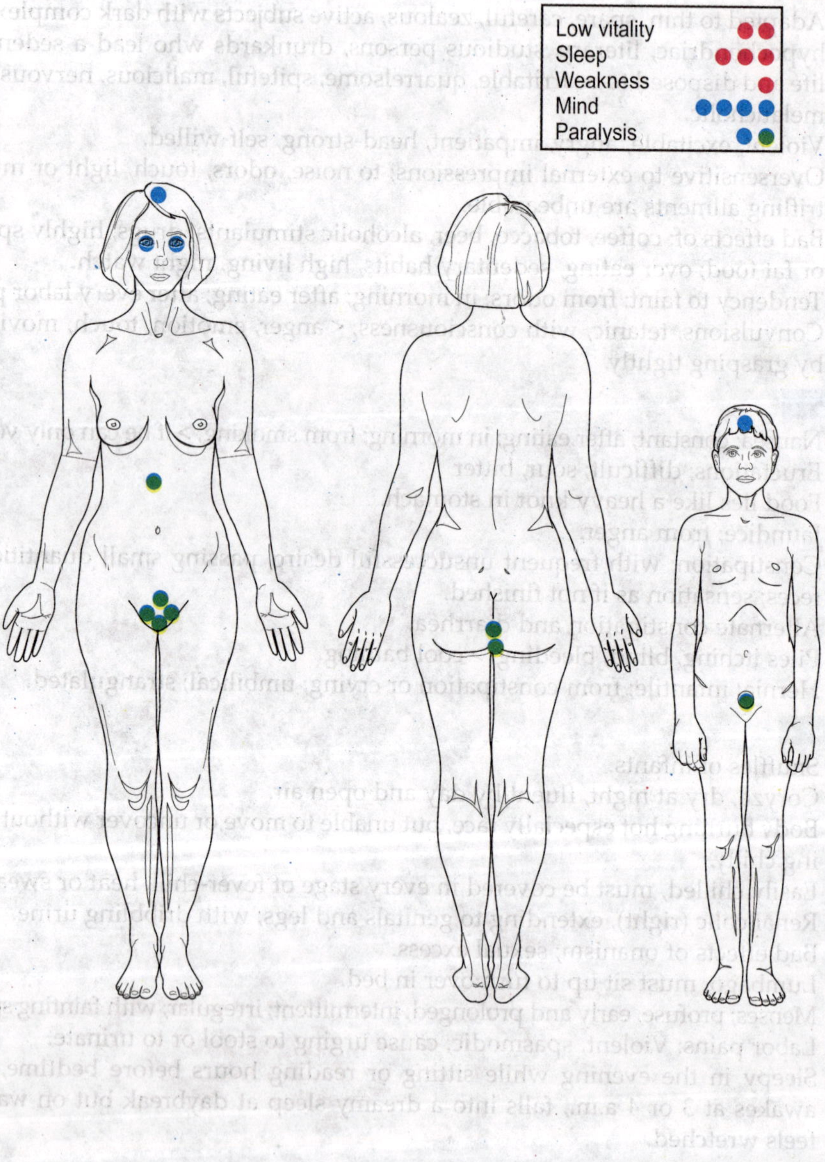

OPIUM

Poppy
Papaveraceae

- Especially adapted to children and old people; diseases of first and second childhood.
- Persons with light hair, lax muscles and want of bodily irritability.
- Child with wrinkled skin, look like a little dried up old man.
- There is want of susceptibility to remedies, lack of vital reaction and the well chosen remedy makes no impression.
- All complaints: with great sopor; painless, complains of nothing; wants nothing.
- Sleep heavy, stupid; with stertorous breathing, red face, eyes half-closed, blood-shot; skin covered with hot sweat.
- Sleepy, but cannot sleep, sleeplessness with acuteness of hearing.
- Insensibility of nerves; painlessness, depression; drowsy stupor; torpidity and general sluggishness of function.
- Loss of power; of concentration; self control, and judgement.
- Delirium: constantly talking, eyes wild open, face red, puffed; or unconscious, eyes glassy, half-closed, face pale, deep coma preceded by stupor.

- Delirium tremens; in old emaciated persons.
- Thinks she is not at home.
- Bed feels so hot she cannot lie on it, moves often in search of a cool place; must be uncovered.
- Picking of bed clothes during sleep.
- Ailments with insensibility and partial or complete paralysis; that originate from fright, bad effects of, the fear still remaining.
- Ill effects of fear, fright, anger, shame, sudden joy; charcoal fumes, sun.
- Epilepsy; in sleep; of children, from approach of strangers; from fright, from crying < glare of light, from anger, insult; eyes half open and upturned.

- Digestive organs inactive: peristaltic motion reversed or paralyzed; bowels seem closed.
- Obstinate constipation; from inaction or paresis, no desire; from lead poisoning; stool hard, round, black balls.
- Stool: involuntary, especially after fright; black and offensive; from paralysis of sphincter.
- Retention of urine: with bladder full; from spasms of neck of bladder; post partum; from excessive use of tobacco; in nursing children, after passion of nurse; from fright; in fever or acute illness.
- Paralytic atony of bladder; after laparotomy.
- Amenorrhoea from fright.
- Threatened abortion, and suppression of lochia from fright.

SURFACE MARKING OF KEYNOTES

PETROLEUM

	Mind	●●
	Skin	●●●●● ●●●●●

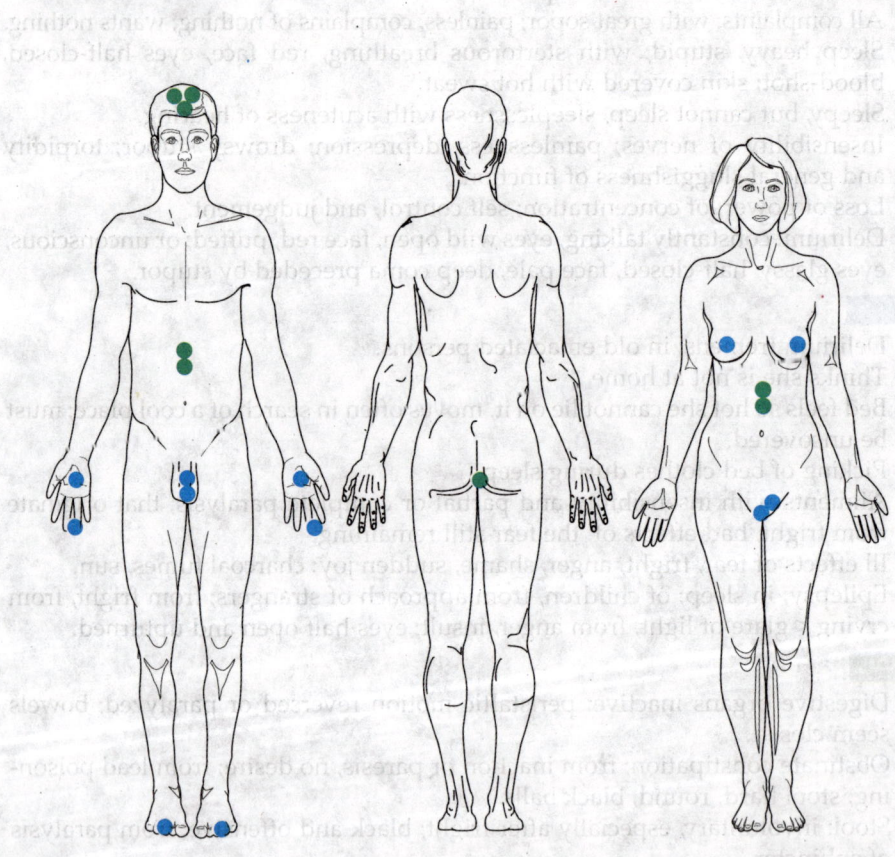

176 P

PETROLEUM

Coal or Rock Oil
Anthracite

- Adapted to lean, emaciated subjects with light hair and skin; irritable, quarrelsome disposition.
- Long lasting, deep seated wasting diseases.
- Ailments; from riding in a carriage; car, train, or in a ship.
- Sense of duality, thinks he is double or some one else lying alongside or one limb is double.
- Easily offended at trifles; vexed at everything.

- Painful sensitiveness of skin of whole body; all clothing is painful; slight injury suppurates.
- Skin: dirty, hard, dry, rough, thickened; leathery, constricted, cracked, fissured.
- Deep cracks; in angles, nipples, finger tips, bleed easily.
- Rough, cracked, fissured hands and tips of fingers, < every winter; > in summer.
- All eruptions itch violently, parts becomes cold after scratching.
- Chilblains that itch, burn and become purple.
- Herpes: of genital organs extending to perineum and thighs.
- Sweat and moisture of external genitals, both sexes.

- Vertigo on rising; in occiput, as if intoxicated; like seasickness.
- Headache: in occiput, which is as heavy as lead.
- Head feels numb as if made of wood.
- Nausea: train and seasickness; during pregnancy, must stoop, in morning.
- Gastralgia: of pregnancy; with pressing, drawing pains; when ever stomach is empty; relieved by constant eating.
- Diarrhea: yellow, watery, gushing; after cabbege, sour fruits; during pregnancy, stormy weather; always in the daytime.

SURFACE MARKING OF KEYNOTES

PHOSPHORUS

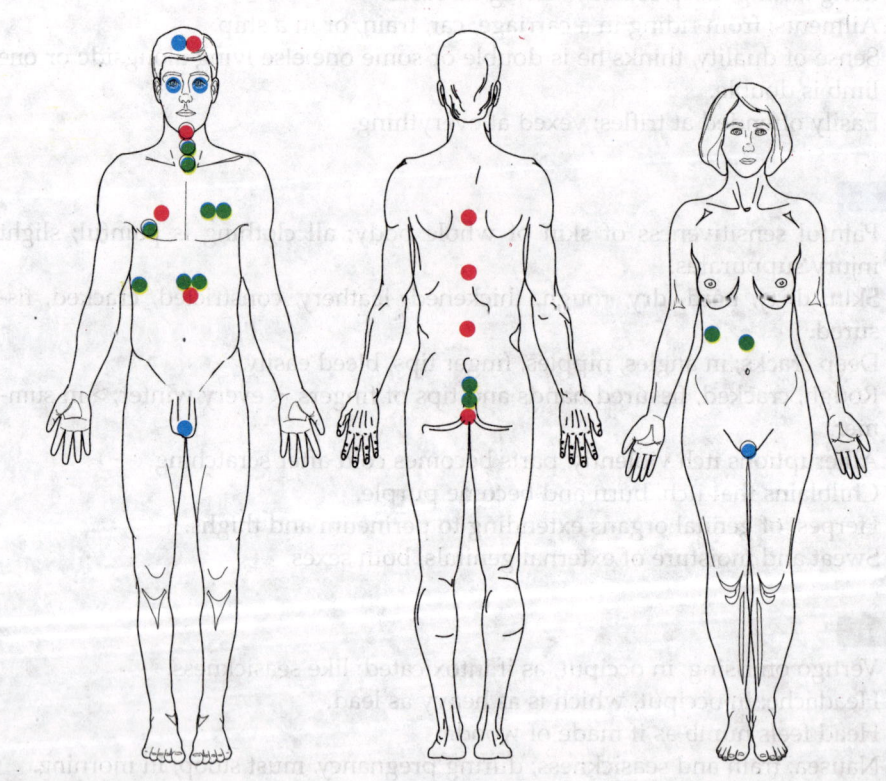

PHOSPHORUS

Phosphorus
P

- Adapted to tall slender persons of sanguine temperament, fair skin, delicate eyelashes, fine blond, or red hair.
- Young people who grow too rapidly are inclined to stoop; who are chlorotic or anemic; old people, with morning diarrhea.
- Nervous, weak, delicate; desires to be magnetized.
- Great weakness and prostration; with nervous debility and trembling from loss of vital fluids.
- Hemorrhages; recurrent, vicarious; small wounds bleed much.
- Burning: in spots along the spine.
- Emptiness; in head, chest, stomach etc.
- Caries; of the bones; spine; lower jaw.

- Over sensitiveness of all the senses to external impressions, light, noise, odors, touch, electrical changes etc.
- Melancholy; disinclined to work, study, converse. Weary of life.
- Anxious, restlessness, cannot sit or stand still for a moment.
- Amative; will uncover his body and expose his genitals.
- Eyes; hollow, surrounded by blue rings; lids, puffy, swollen, oedematous.
- Dandruff, falls out in clouds; hair falls out in bunches of single spots.

- Craves cold food and drinks; which > but are vomited in a little while, when it becomes warm in the stomach.
- Nausea from placing hands in warm water.
- During pregnancy; unable to drink water; sight of it causes vomiting; must close her eyes while bathing.
- Constipation: feces slender, long, dry, tough and hard.
- Diarrhea: as soon as anything enters the rectum; profuse watery with sago-like particles; sensation, as if the anus remained open involuntary; morning, of old people.
- Jaundice; with pneumonia or brain disease; during pregnancy; malignant.
- Pain; in intercostal spaces; excited by slightest chill; < from slightest pressure, lying on left side, open air.
- Larynx; painful, dry, raw, rough, sore.
- Cough: going from warm to cold air; < from laughing, talking, reading, drinking, eating, lying on left side.
- Pneumonia; of left lower lung.
- Haemoptysis. Tuberculosis.

SURFACE MARKING OF KEYNOTES

PHYTOLACCA DECANDRA

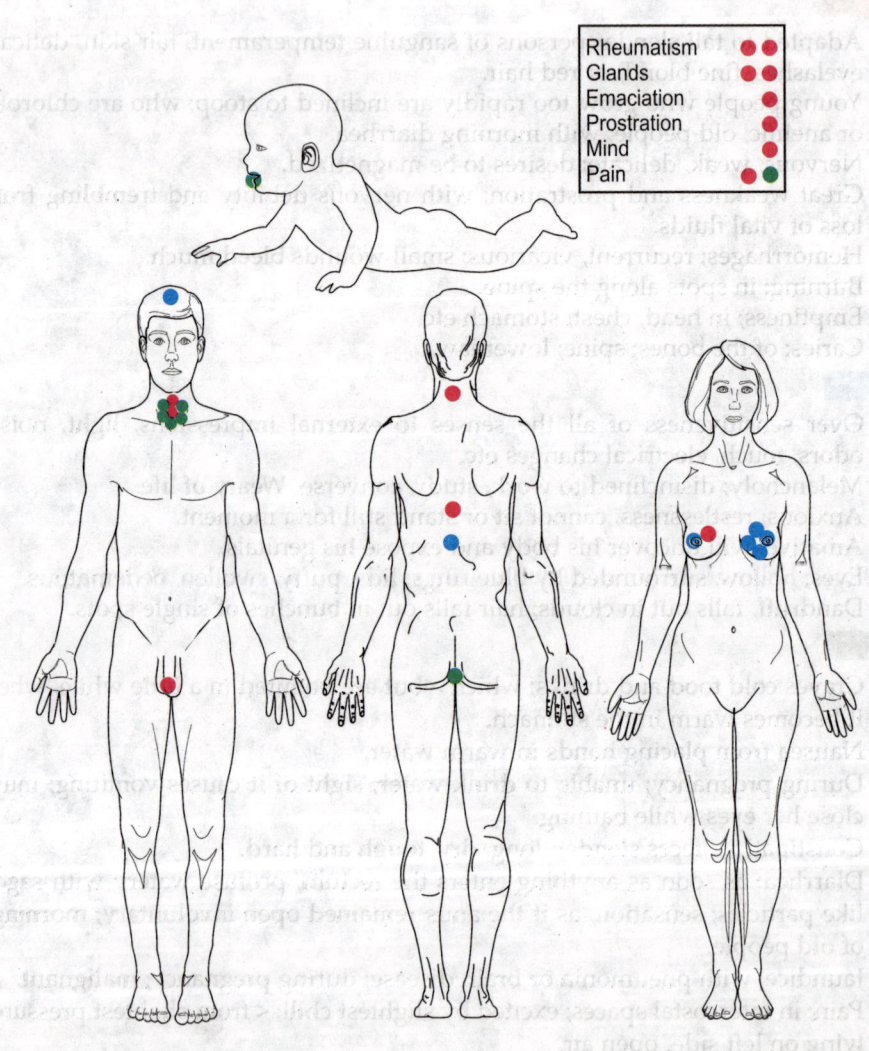

180 P

PHYTOLACCA DECANDRA

Poke Root
Phytolaccaceae

- Patients of rheumatic diathesis; rheumatism of fibrous and periosteal tissue.
- Affects the glands especially mammary and tonsils; muscle of neck and back.
- Emaciation, chlorosis; loss of fat.
- Great exhaustion and profound prostration.
- Entire indifference to life; sure she will die.
- Pain flying like electric shocks; shooting, lancinating; rapidly shifting; worse from motion and at night.
- In rheumatism and neuralgia after diphtheria, gonorrhea, mercury or syphilis.

- Intense headache and backache; lame, sore, bruised feeling all over; constant desire to move but motion < pains.
- Mammae full of hard, painful nodosities.
- Breast, shows an early tendency to cake; is full, heavy, stony, hard and painful.
- Mammary abscess; fistula, gaping, angry ulcers; pus sanious, ihorous, fetid; unhealthy.
- Nipples, sensitive, sore fissured; inverted.
- When child nurses pain goes from nipple all over body.

- Irresistible desire to bite the teeth or gums together; during dentition.
- Sore throat; of a dark red or bluished red colour; very painful on swallowing; dryness; burning as from a coal of fire or a red-hot iron.
- Pains shoot from throat into ears on swallowing.
- Sensation of a lump in the throat with continuous desire to swallow.
- Cannot swallow anything hot.
- Tonsillitis. Diphtheria.
- Dysentery; passage only of mucus and blood or like scraping from the intestines.

SURFACE MARKING OF KEYNOTES

PLATINUM METALLICUM

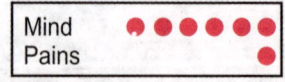

182 P

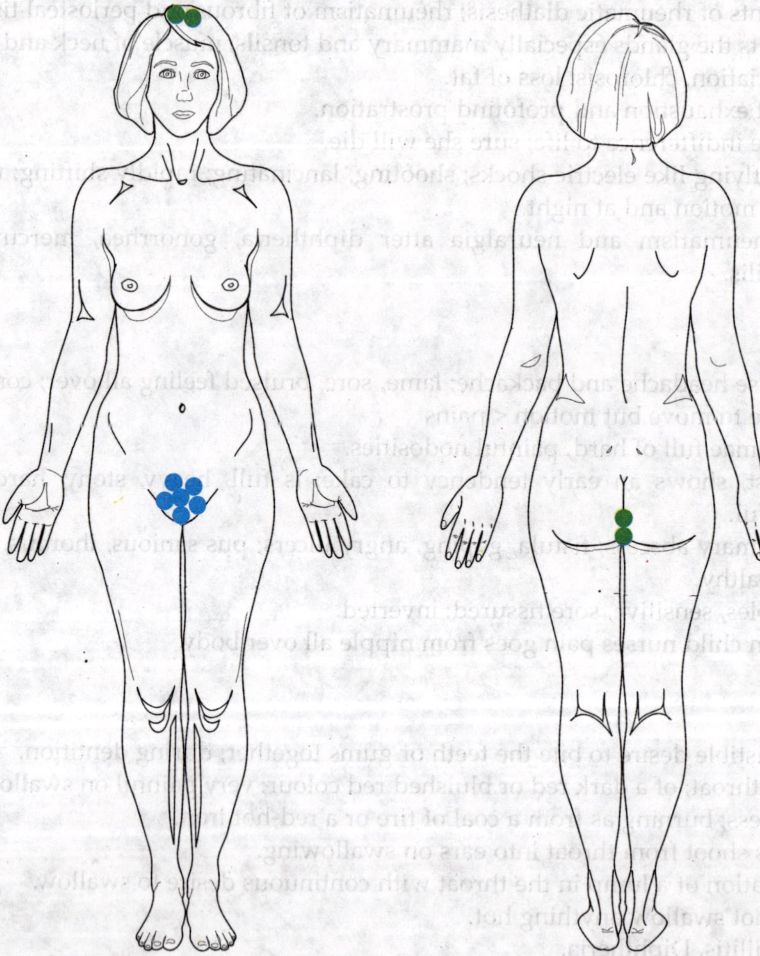

PLATINUM METALLICUM

Platina
Pt

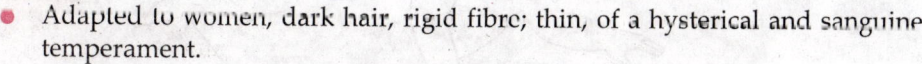

- Adapted to women, dark hair, rigid fibre; thin, of a hysterical and sanguine temperament.
- Mental disturbances after fright, grief, vexation; onanism, pride.
- Arrogant, proud, contemptuous, and haughty.
- Mental delusions, as if everything about her were small; all persons physically and mentally inferior, but she is physically large and superior.
- Sensation of growing larger in every direction.
- Alternate mental and physical or sexual symptoms.
- Satiety of life, with taciturnity and fear of death.
- The pains increase gradually and as gradually decrease; are attended with numbness of parts.

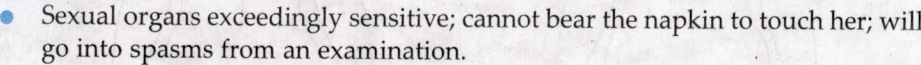

- Sexual organs exceedingly sensitive; cannot bear the napkin to touch her; will go into spasms from an examination.
- Vulva painfully sensitive during coitus; will faint during, or cannot endure, coitus. Vaginismus.
- Nymphomania; < in lying-in women.
- Excessive sexual desire especially in virgins; that leads to masturbation.
- Pruritis vulvae; with voluptuous tingling.
- Menses too early, too profuse, too long-lasting; dark-clotted, offensive, with bearing down spasms.

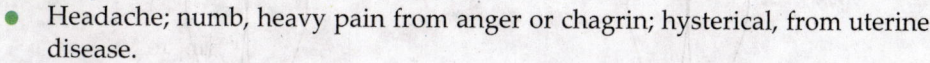

- Headache; numb, heavy pain from anger or chagrin; hysterical, from uterine disease.
- Epilepsy; catalepsy.
- Constipation; while travelling; after lead poisoning; of emigrants; of pregnancy.
- Constipation: from inertia of bowels; frequent, unsuccessful urging; stools adhere to rectum and anus like soft clay.

SURFACE MARKING OF KEYNOTES

PODOPHYLLUM

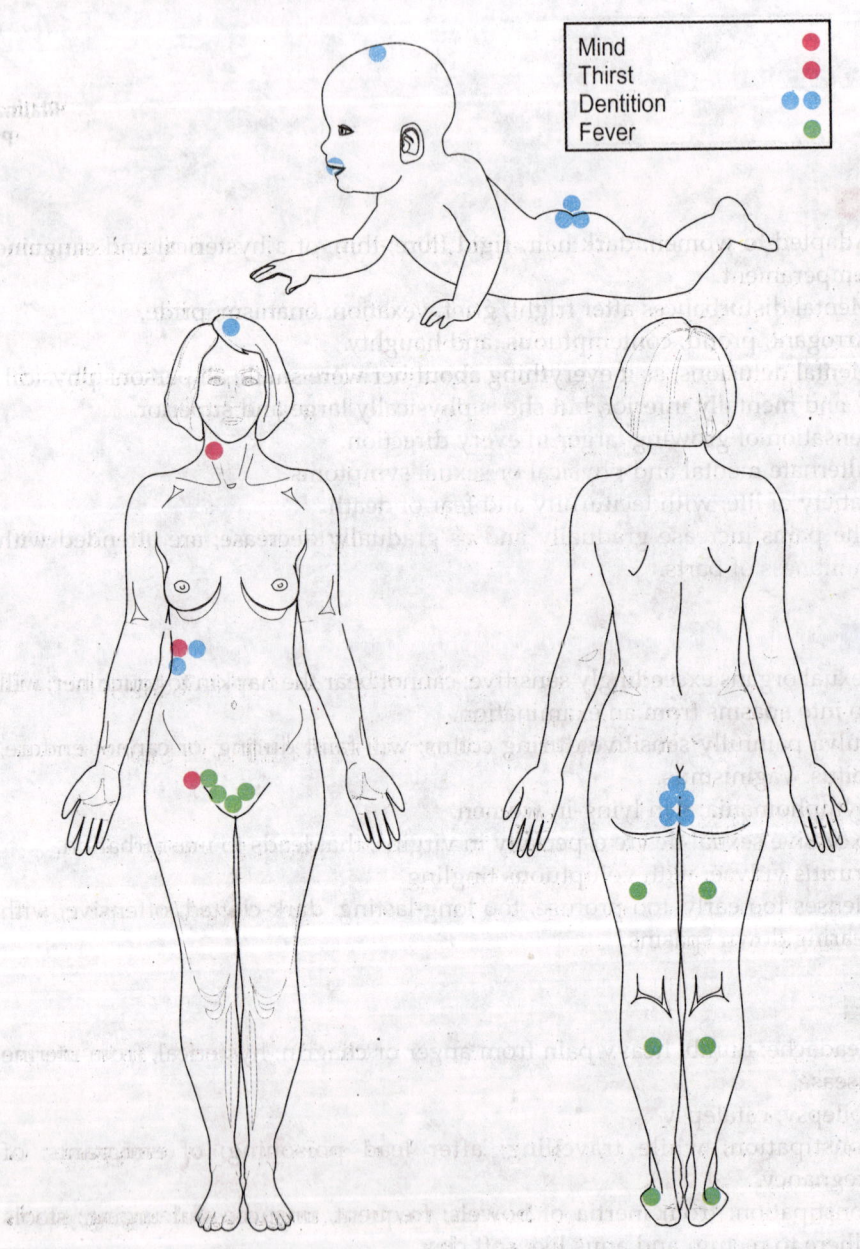

PODOPHYLLUM

May Apple
Berberidaceae

- Adapted to persons of bilious temperament who suffer from gastro-intestinal derangement, especially after abuse of mercury.
- Affects right throat, right ovary, right hypochondrium.
- Depression of spirits, imagines he is going to die or be very ill; disgust for life.
- Thirst for large quantities of cold water.

- Difficult dentition: moaning, grinding the teeth at night; intense desire to press the gums together; head hot and rolling from side to side.
- Patient is constantly rubbing and shaking the region of liver with his hand.
- Jaundice, with gall-stones.
- Painless cholera morbus; cholera infantum.
- Diarrhea: of long standing; early in morning, continues through forenoon, followed by natural stool in evening.
- Diarrhea of children: during teething; after eating; while being bathed or washed; of dirty water socking napkin through; with gagging.
- Stool: green, watery, foetid, profuse; gushing out.
- Prolapse of rectum; before or with stool, from debility of childhood, after parturition, during pregnancy.
- Headache alternates with diarrhea; headache in winter, diarrhea in summer.

- Violent cramps in feet, calves; thighs; with watery, painless stools.
- Prolapsus uteri: from overlifting or straining; from constipation; after parturition; with subinvolution.
- In early months of pregnancy, can lie comfortably only on stomach.
- Pain and numbness in right ovary, running down thigh of that side, < stretching the legs.
- Suppressed menses in young girls.
- Fever paroxysm at 7 a.m. with great loquacity during chill and heat; sleep during perspiration.

SURFACE MARKING OF KEYNOTES

PULSATILLA

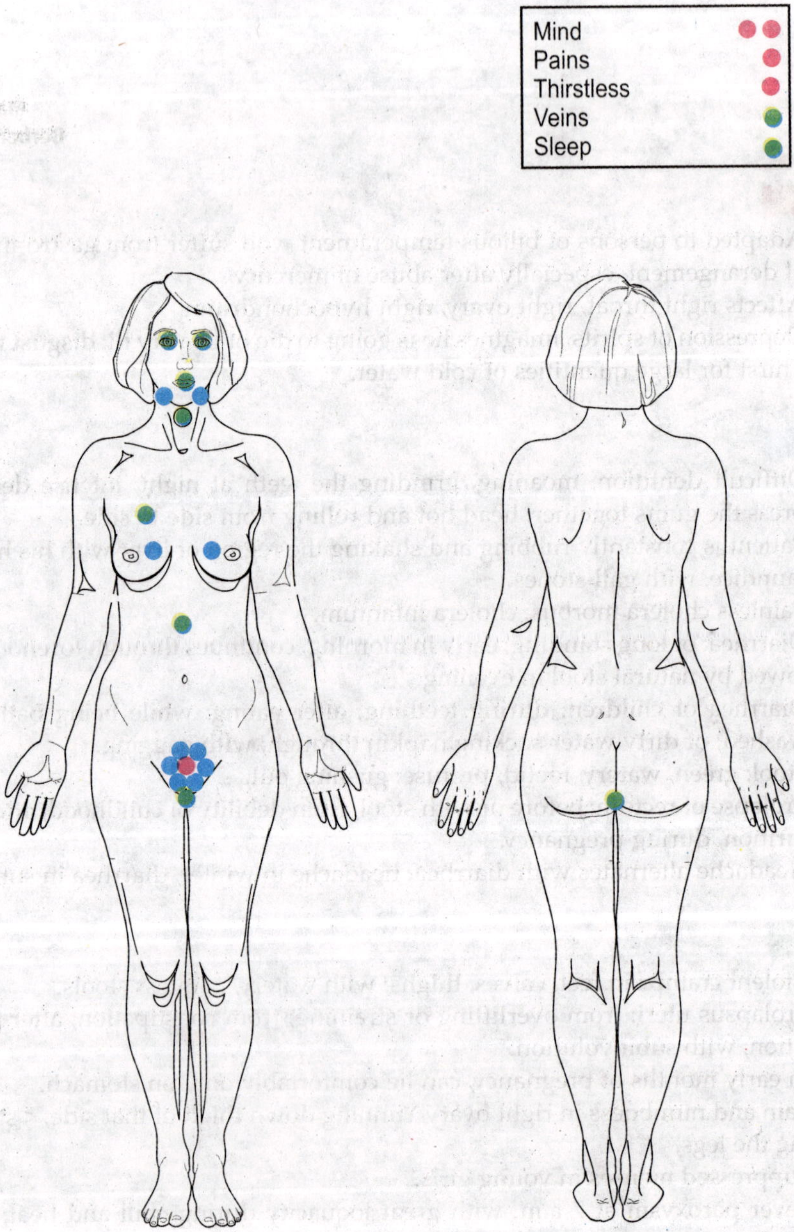

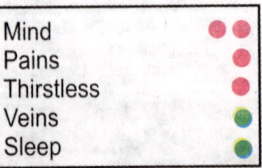

Mind
Pains
Thirstless
Veins
Sleep

186 P

PULSATILLA

Anemone
Ranunculaceae

- Adapted to persons of indecisive, slow, phlegmatic temperament; sandy hair, blue eyes, pale face, affectionate, mild, gentle, timid yielding disposition - the woman's remedy.
- Women inclined to be fleshy, with scanty and protracted menstruation.
- Weeps easily: almost impossible to detail her ailments without weeping > by consolation.
- Symptoms ever changing; no two chills, no two stools, no two attacks alike.
- Pains: rapidly shifting from one part to another; are accompanied with constant chilliness; the more severe the pain, the more severe the chill; appear suddenly, leave gradually.
- Secretions from all mucous membranes are thick bland and yellowish-green.
- Thirstlessness with nearly all complaints.

- Derangements at puberty.
- Delayed first menstruation.
- Menses, suppressed from getting the feet wet.
- Menses too late, scanty, slimy, painful, irregular, intermittent flow with evening chilliness; flows more during day.
- Dysmenorrhoea with great restlessness and tossing about.
- Threatened abortion; flow ceases and then returns with increased force.
- Maldisposition of foetus.
- Mumps; metastasis to mammae or testicles.

- Styes: especially on upper lid; from eating fat, greasy, rich food or pork; recurrent.
- Toothache; > by holding cold water in the mouth; < from warm things and heat of room.
- Gastric difficulties from eating rich food, cake, pastry, especially after pork or sausage.
- Diarrhea: only, or usually at night; watery, greenish-yellow, very changeable; soon as they eat; from fruit, cold food or drinks, ice-cream.
- Bronchitis, phthisis in chlorotic and anemic girls.
- Cough after measles.
- Veins full, varicose, painful.
- Thick yellow discharge, late stage of gonorrhea.
- Great sleepiness during day, wakes confused; languid, unrefreshed.

SURFACE MARKING OF KEYNOTES

RHUS TOXICODENDRON

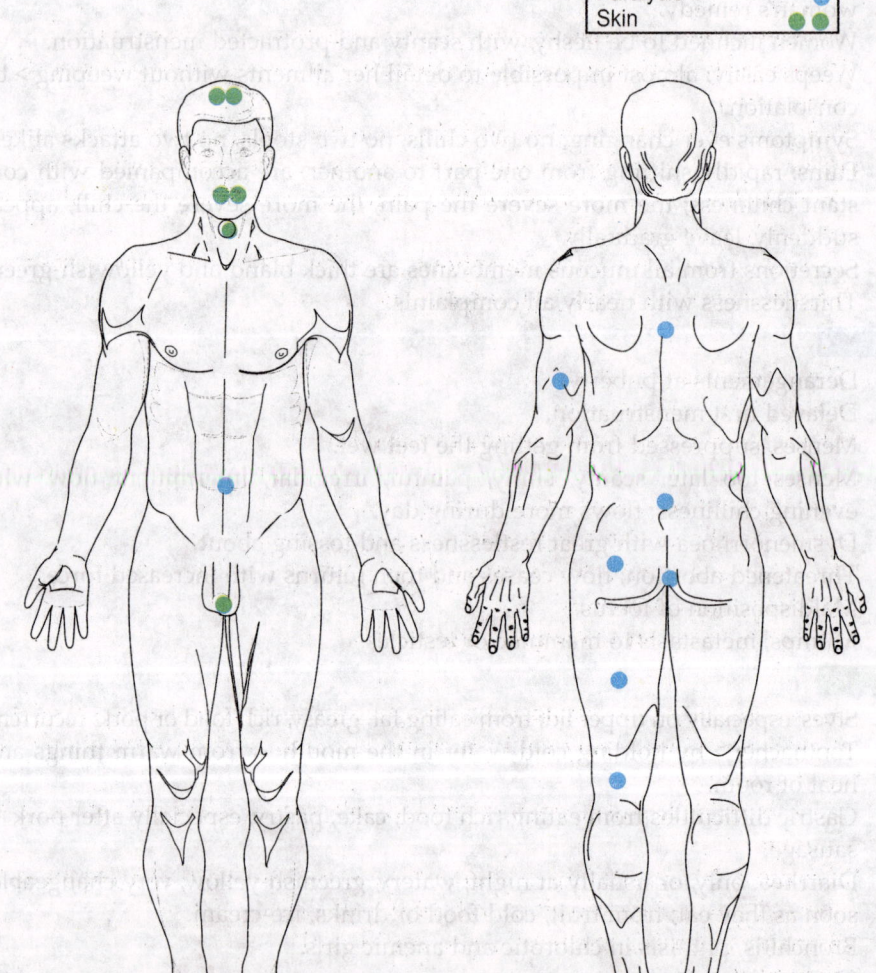

188 R

RHUS TOXICODENDRON

Poison Oak
Anacardiaceae

- Adapted to persons of rheumatic diathesis, affects the fibrous tissue.
- Ailments: from spraining or straining a single part, muscle or tendon; over-lifting; too much summer bathing in lake or river.
- Bad effects of getting wet, especially after being over-heated.
- Great restlessness, anxiety, apprehension; cannot remain in bed, must change position often to obtain relief from pain.
- Great thirst, with dry tongue, mouth and throat.

- Pains: as if sprained; as if a muscle or tendon was torn from its attachment; as if bones were scraped with a knife; worse after midnight and in wet, rainy weather; affected parts sore to touch.
- Lameness, stiffness and pain on first moving after rest, on getting up in the morning, > by walking or continued motion.
- Back: pain between the shoulders on swallowing; pain and stiffness in small of back.
- Muscular rheumatism, sciatica, left side; aching in left arm, with heart disease.
- Paralysis: with numbness of affected parts; from getting wet on lying on damp ground; after exertion, parturition, sexual excesses, ague or typhoid.
- Diarrhea: with beginning typhoid; involuntary, with great exhaustion; tearing pain down the posterior part of limbs during stool.
- When acute diseases assume a typhoid form.

- Vertigo, when standing or walking; worse when lying down.
- Headache: brain feels loose when stepping or shaking the head; from beer; > warmth and motion.
- Corners of mouth ulcerated, fever blisters around mouth and on chin.
- Tongue: dry, sore, red, cracked; triangular red tip; takes imprint of teeth.
- A dry, teasing cough, before and during chill, in intermittent fever.
- External genitals inflamed, erysipelatous, oedematous.
- Erysipelas, from left to right; vesicular, yellow vesicles; much swelling, inflammation; burning; itching, stinging.

SURFACE MARKING OF KEYNOTES

SECALE CORNUTUM

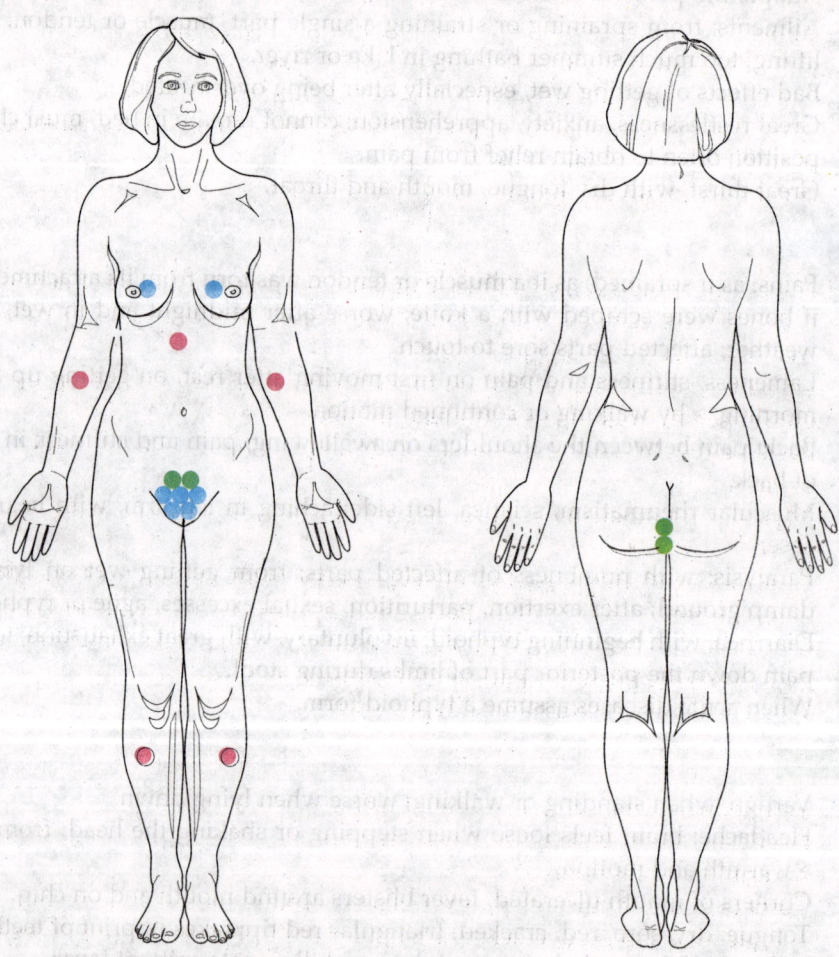

Prostration
Haemorrhage
Skin

SECALE CORNUTUM

Spurred Rye; Ergot
A Fungus; A Nosode

- Adapted to women of thin, scrawny, feeble, cachectic appearance, irritable, nervous temperament; pale, sunken countenance.
- Very old, decrepit, feeble persons.
- Women of very lax muscular fibre; everything seems loose and open; no action; vessels flabby.
- Hemorrhagic diathesis; the slightest wound causes bleeding for weeks.
- Passive hemorrhages, copious flow of thin, black, watery blood; the corpuscles are destroyed.
- The skin feels cold to the touch, yet the patient cannot tolerate covering; icy coldness of extremities.
- Burning; in all parts of the body; as if sparks of fire were falling on the patient.
- Unnatural, ravenous appetite; even with exhausting diarrhea.

- Menses: irregular; copious; dark fluid; continuous discharge of watery blood until next period.
- Leucorrhoea; green, brown, offensive.
- Threatened abortion especially at third month; prolonged, bearing down, forcing pains.
- During labor: pains irregular; too weak; feeble or ceasing; everything seems loose and open but to expulsive action; fainting.
- After pains: too long; too painful; hour-glass contraction.
- Suppression of milk; the breasts do not properly fill.

- Boils; small, painful with green contents, mature very slowly and heal in the same manner; very debilitating.
- Gangrene; dry senile, < from external heat.
- Large ecchymosis; blood blisters.
- Pulse small, rapid, contracted and often intermittent.
- Diarrhea: profuse, watery, putrid, brown; discharged with great force; very exhausting; painless; involuntary; anus wide open.
- Collapse in cholera diseases.
- Enuresis of old people.
- Urine pale, watery, or bloody; suppressed.

SURFACE MARKING OF KEYNOTES

SEPIA

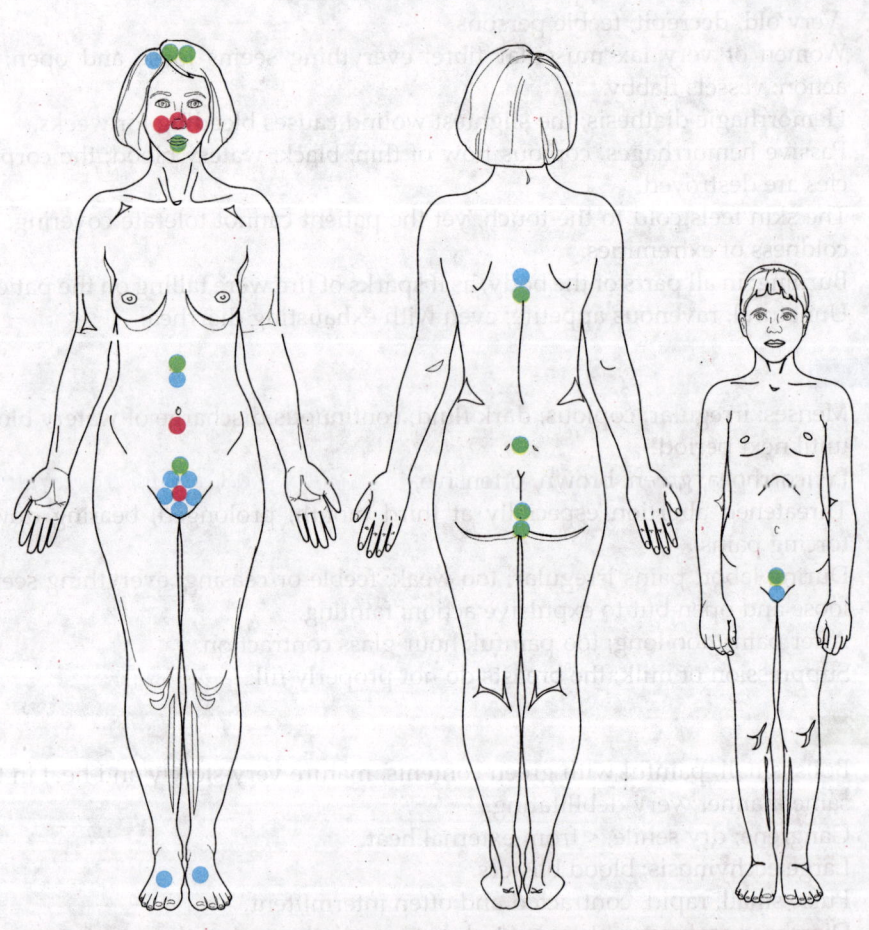

SEPIA

Cuttle Fish
Mollusca

- Adapted to persons of dark hair, rigid fibre, but mild and easy disposition.
- Diseases of women: especially those occurring during pregnancy; childbed and lactation.
- Weak, pot-bellied mothers with yellow complexion.
- A yellow saddle across upper part of the cheeks and nose.
- The washer woman's remedy, complaints that are brought on by or aggravated after laundry work.
- Diseases attended with sudden prostration and sinking faintness.
- Sensation of a ball in inner parts.
- Flushes of heat from least motion; with anxiety and faintness; climacteric; ascends, from pelvic organs.
- Great sadness and weeping. Dread of being alone, of men; of meeting friends; with uterine troubles.
- Indifferent: even to one's family; to one's occupation; to those whom she loves best.
- Indolent: does not want to do anything, either work or play.

- Prolapsus of uterus and vagina; pressure and bearing down as if everything would protrude from pelvis; must cross limbs tightly or "sit close" to prevent it.
- Irregular menses of nearly every form—early, late, scanty, profuse, amenorrhea or menorrhagia.
- Leucorrhoea: yellow, greenish, milky, in large lumps, in little girls; instead of menses, foul; gonorrheal.
- Aversion to coition, or complaints after.
- Tendency to abortion; from 5th to 7th month.
- Nausea; at thought or smell of food; in morning; thought of coition, during pregnancy.
- Cold; in spots; on vertex; between scapulae; feet, in bed.

- Headache: in terrific shocks; at menstrual period with scanty flow; in delicate, sensitive, hysterical women.
- Great falling of the hair, after chronic headaches or at the climacteric.
- Tongue dirty, becomes clear during menses.
- Painful sensation of emptiness, "All-gone feeling", in the epigastrium, relieved by eating.
- Constipation: during pregnancy; stool hard, knotty, in balls, insufficient, difficult.
- Sense of weight or ball in anus, not > by stool.
- Urine; thick, foul; white gritty or adherent red sandy sediment.
- Enuresis: bed is wet almost as soon as the child goes to sleep; always during the first sleep.
- Aching in inter-scapular or lumbar region; paralytic; wants to be pressed.
- Itching of skin; of various parts; of external genitalia; is not > by scratching.
- Herpes circinatus in isolated spots on upper part of body.

SURFACE MARKING OF KEYNOTES

SILICEA

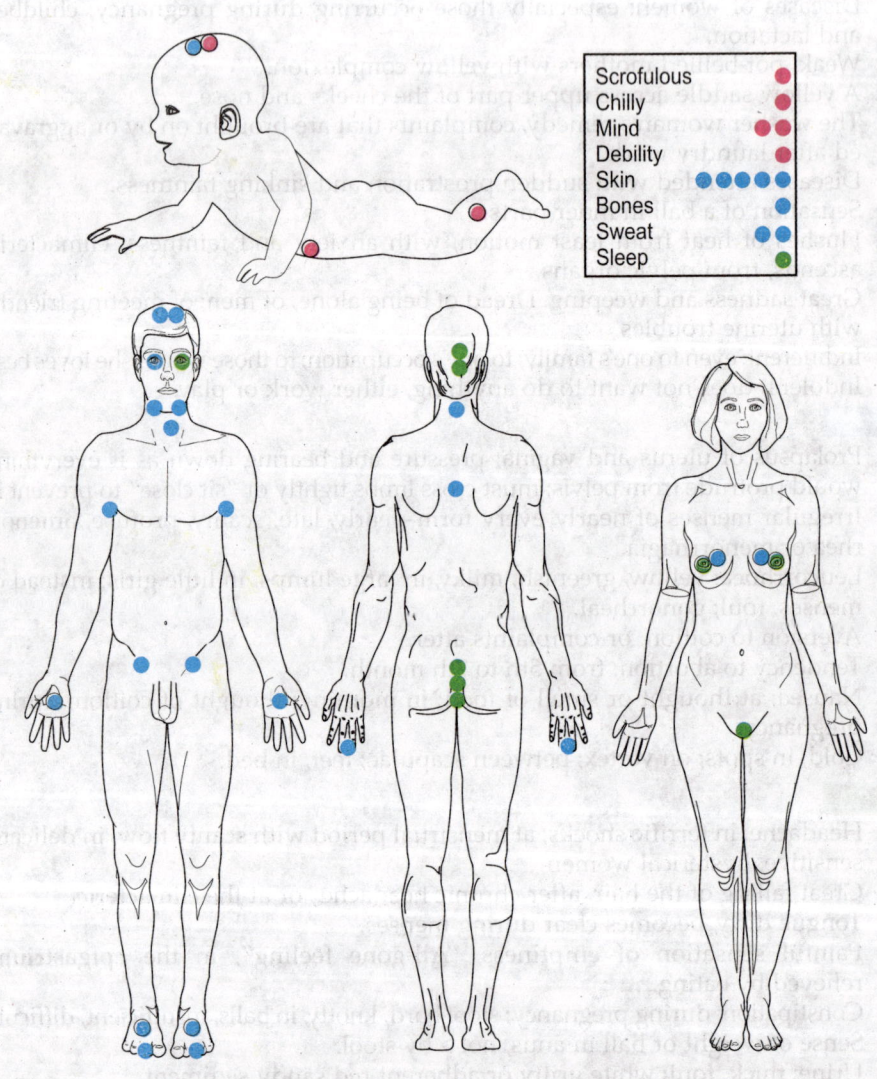

Scrofulous	●
Chilly	● ●
Mind	● ●
Debility	●
Skin	● ● ● ● ● ●
Bones	● ● ●
Sweat	● ●
Sleep	●

SILICEA

Pure Silica
SiO_2

- It is best suited to persons with pale face, lean and thin body, weak and lax musculature, sickly appearance with dry skin.
- Person whose assimilation is imperfect and consequently suffer from defective nutrition.
- Scrofulous, rachitic children with large head, open fontanelles and sutures, distended abdomen, slow walking, who are obstinate and head strong.
- Want of vital heat, always chilly, even when taking active exercise.
- Restless fidgety, starts at least noise.
- Anxious, yielding, fainthearted, mental labor very difficult.
- Great weariness and debility; wants to lie down.

- Ailments: caused by suppressed foot-sweat; stone cutting; exposing the head or back to any slight draft of air; bad effects of vaccination, especially abscesses and convulsions.
- Inflammation, swelling and suppuration of glands, tonsils, cervical, axillary, parotid, mammary, inguinal, sebaceous, malignant, gangrenous.
- Unhealthy skin; every little injury suppurates.
- Fistula lachrymalis: fistulae, painful, offensive, high spongy edges, proud flesh in them.
- Panaritium; blood boils; carbuncles; elephantiasis, ulcers of all kinds.
- Promotes expulsion of foreign bodies from the tissues; fish bones, needles, bone splinters.
- Diseases of bones and cartilages; caries and necrosis; softening of bones.
- Sweat of head, hands, toes, feet and axillae; offensive, profuse.

- Vertigo; ascends from dorsal region < looking upwards, closing eyes.
- Chronic sick headache, since some severe disease of youth; ascending from nape of neck to the vertex, < draft of air or uncovering the head, while fasting; > pressure and wrapping up warmly.
- Cataract in office workers.
- Constipation: always before and during menses; difficult as from inactivity of rectum; with great straining, as if rectum was paralyzed; when partly expelled, recedes again.
- Fistula in ano alternates with chest symptoms.
- Fissura ani; great pain after stool.
- Bloody discharge from vagina < nursing; between periods.
- Nipple is drawn in like a funnel.
- Night walking; gets up while asleep, walks about and lies down again.

SURFACE MARKING OF KEYNOTES

SPONGIA TOSTA

Scrofulous	●
Tubercular	●
Sleep	●
Exhaustion	●

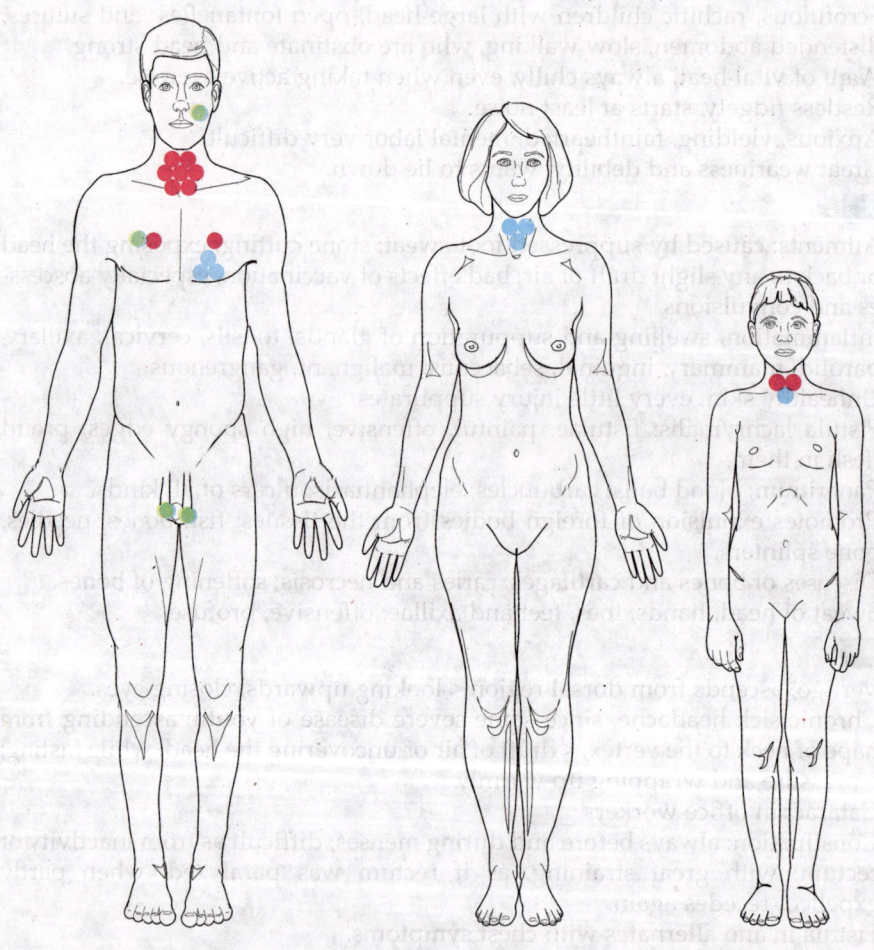

SPONGIA TOSTA

Roasted sponge
Poosifera

- Especially adapted to diseases of children and women; light hair, lax fibre, fair complexion, flabby and scrofulous constitutions, and the tubercular diathesis.
- Great dryness of mucous membranes of air passages - throat, larynx, trachea, bronchi - "dry as a horn".
- Cough dry, barking, croupy; rasping, ringing, wheezing, whistling; everything is perfectly dry, no mucus rale.
- Cough: dry, sibilant, like a saw driven through a pine board; < sweets, cold drinks, smoking, lying with head low, dry cold winds; < reading, singing, talking, swallowing; > eating or drinking warm things.
- Every mental excitement < or increase the cough.
- Croup: anxious, wheezing, < during inspiration; < before midnight.
- Awakens in a fright and feels as if suffocating; as if he had to breath through a sponge.

- Swelling and induration of glands.
- Thyroid gland swollen; even with the chin.
- Goitre; with suffocative spells; < pressure.
- Sore throat, < after eating sweet things.
- Worse after sleep or sleeps into.
- Palpitation: violent with pain and gasping respiration; valvular insufficiency; before or during menses.
- Angina pectoris; contracting pain, heat, faintness, suffocation, anxiety and sweat; < after midnight.
- Hypertrophy of heart with asthmatic symptoms.

- Exhaustion and heaviness of the body, with slight exertion; must lie down; with orgasm of blood to chest, face etc.
- Painful swelling of spermatic cord and testicles.

SURFACE MARKING OF KEYNOTES

SULPHUR

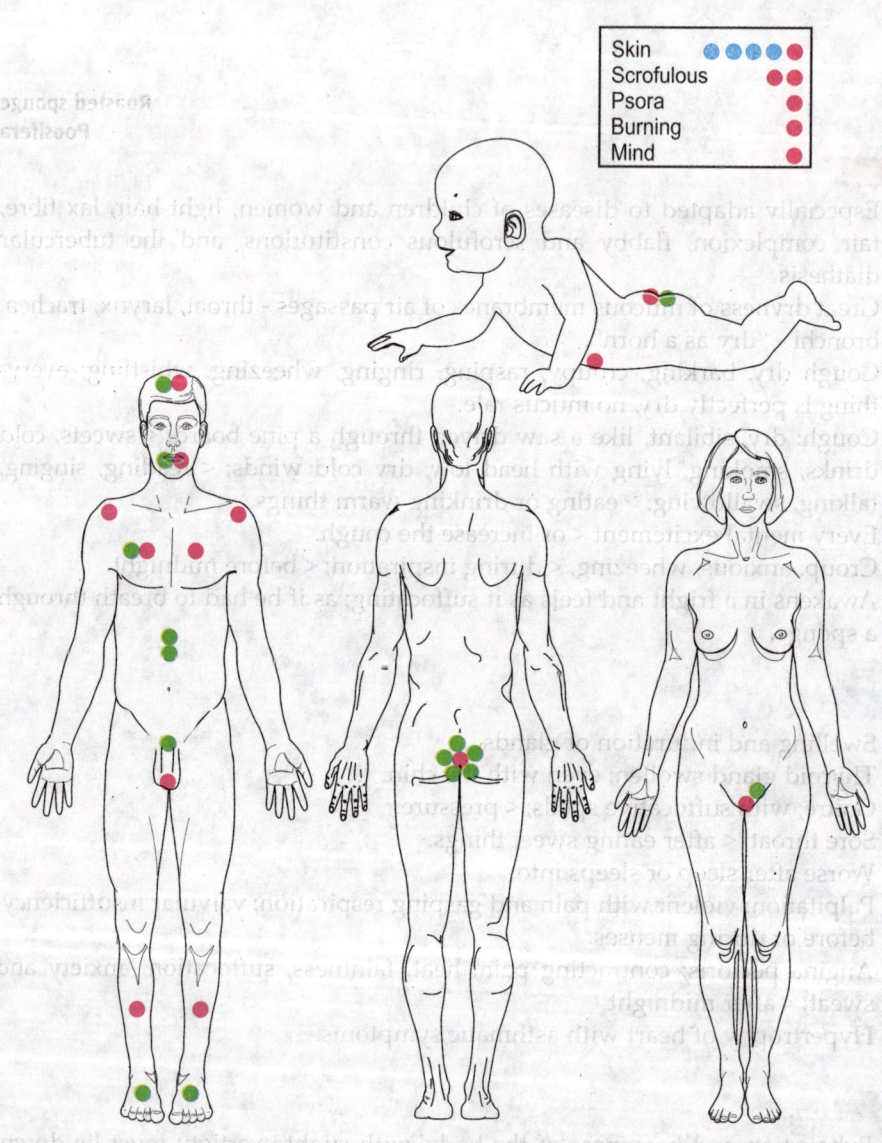

198 S

SULPHUR

Brimstone; Flowers of Sulphur

- For lean, thin, stoop-shouldered persons who walk and sit stooping; walk stooping like old men.
- Standing is the worst position for Sulphur patients.
- Dirty, filthy people, prone to skin affections.
- Persons of nervous temperament, quick motioned, quick tempered, plethoric.
- Persons of scrofulous diathesis, subject to venous congestion; especially of portal system.
- Children: cannot bear to be washed or bathed; emaciated, big-bellied; restless, hot, kick off the clothes at night; have worms.
- Complaints that are continually relapsing.
- When carefully selected remedies fail to produce a favorable effect, especially in acute disease.
- Scrofulous, psoric, chronic disease that result from suppressed emotions.
- Sensation of burning in affected parts.
- Dull difficult thinking; lazy hungry, and always tired, hopeful dreamers.

- All the orifices of the body are very red; all discharges acrid, excoriating wherever they touch.
- Facilitate absorption of serous or inflammatory exudates in brain, pleura, lungs, joints.
- Chronic alcoholism; dropsy and other ailments of drunkards.
- Congestion to single parts; marking the onset of tumors or malignant growths, especially at climacteric.
- Skin; dry, rough; wrinkled, scaly.
- Itching; voluptuous; violent, < at night; in bed; scratching and washing.
- Crops of boils.

- Sick headache every week or every two weeks; prostrating, weakening; with hot vertex and cold feet.
- Bright redness of lips as if the blood would burst through.
- Weak, empty, gone or faint feeling in the stomach about 11 a.m.; cannot wait for lunch.
- Frequent weak, faint spells during the day.
- Diarrhea: after midnight; foul; watery; painful; hurried; driving out of bed early in the morning, < milk.
- Constipation: stools hard, knotty, dry as if burnt; large, painful, child is afraid to have the stool on account of pain.
- The discharge both of urine and faeces is painful to parts over which it passes.
- Parts around anus red, excoriated.
- Piles sore, tender, raw, burn, bleed and smart.
- Menses; irregular, too late, short, scanty, thick, foul, black, acrid, making parts sore.
- Nightly suffocative attacks, wants the doors and windows open.
- Cold feet in daytime with burning soles at night.

SURFACE MARKING OF KEYNOTES

THUJA OCCIDENTALIS

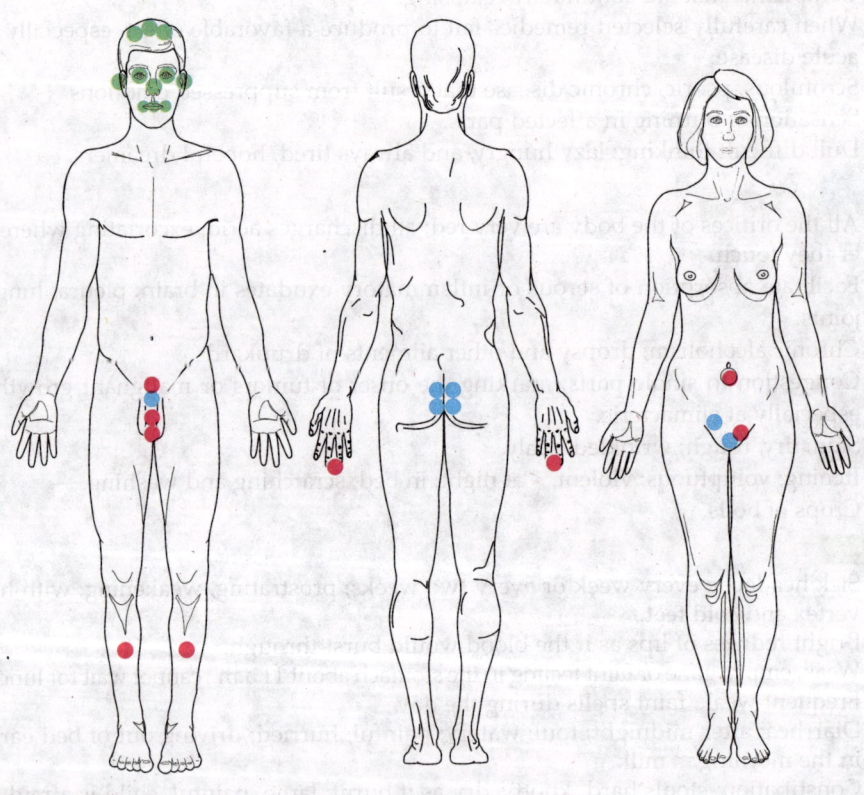

SURFACE MARKING OF KEYNOTES

THUJA OCCIDENTALIS

Tree of life; White Cedar
Coniferae

- Especially adapted to hydrogenoid constitution of Grauvogl, very fleshy persons having dark complexion, black hair, unhealthy, oily, greasy skin.
- Ailments from bad effects of vaccination; from suppressed or maltreated gonorrhea.
- Suppressed gonorrhea: causing articular rheumatism; prostatitis; sycosis; impotence, and condylomata and many constitutional troubles.
- Fixed ideas: as if a strange person were at his side; as if soul and body were separated; as if a living animal were in abdomen; of being under the influence of a superior power.
- Sensation as if body, especially the limbs, were made of glass and would break easily.
- Skin: looks dirty; brown or brownis—white spots here and there.
- Warts, large, seedy, pedunculated.
- Eruptions only on covered parts, burn after scratching.
- Nails: deformed, brittle.
- Sweat; only on uncovered parts; or all over except the head; when he sleeps, stops when he wakes; profuse, sour smelling, fetid, at night; profuse on genitals.

- Constipation: stool recedes, after being partly expelled.
- Piles swollen, pain most severe when sitting.
- Diarrhea; early morning; with much flatus; gurgling, < after breakfast, coffee, fat food, vaccination, onions.
- Anus fissured, painful to touch, surrounded with flat warts, or moist mucus condylomata.
- Sensation after urinating, as of urine trickling in urethra; severe cutting at close of urination.
- Left ovary inflamed, with tearing pain < menses, walking.
- Coition prevented by extreme sensitiveness of the vagina.

- Vertigo, when closing the eyes.
- Headache: as if a nail had been driven into parietal bone; < from sexual excesses; over heating; from tea.
- White scaly dandruff; hair dry and falling out.
- Eyes: ophthalmia neonatorum, large granulations, like warts or blisters; > by warmth and covering.
- Eyelids; agglutinated at night, dry, scaly on edges; styes and tarsal tumors.
- Otorrhoea; watery, purulent; putrid.
- Chronic nasal catarrh: thick, green mucus; blood and pus.
- Teeth decay at the roots, crowns remain sound; crumble, turn yellow.
- Toothache from tea drinking.
- Ranula: bluish, or varicose veins on tongue or in mouth.

T 201

SURFACE MARKING OF KEYNOTES
VERATRUM ALBUM

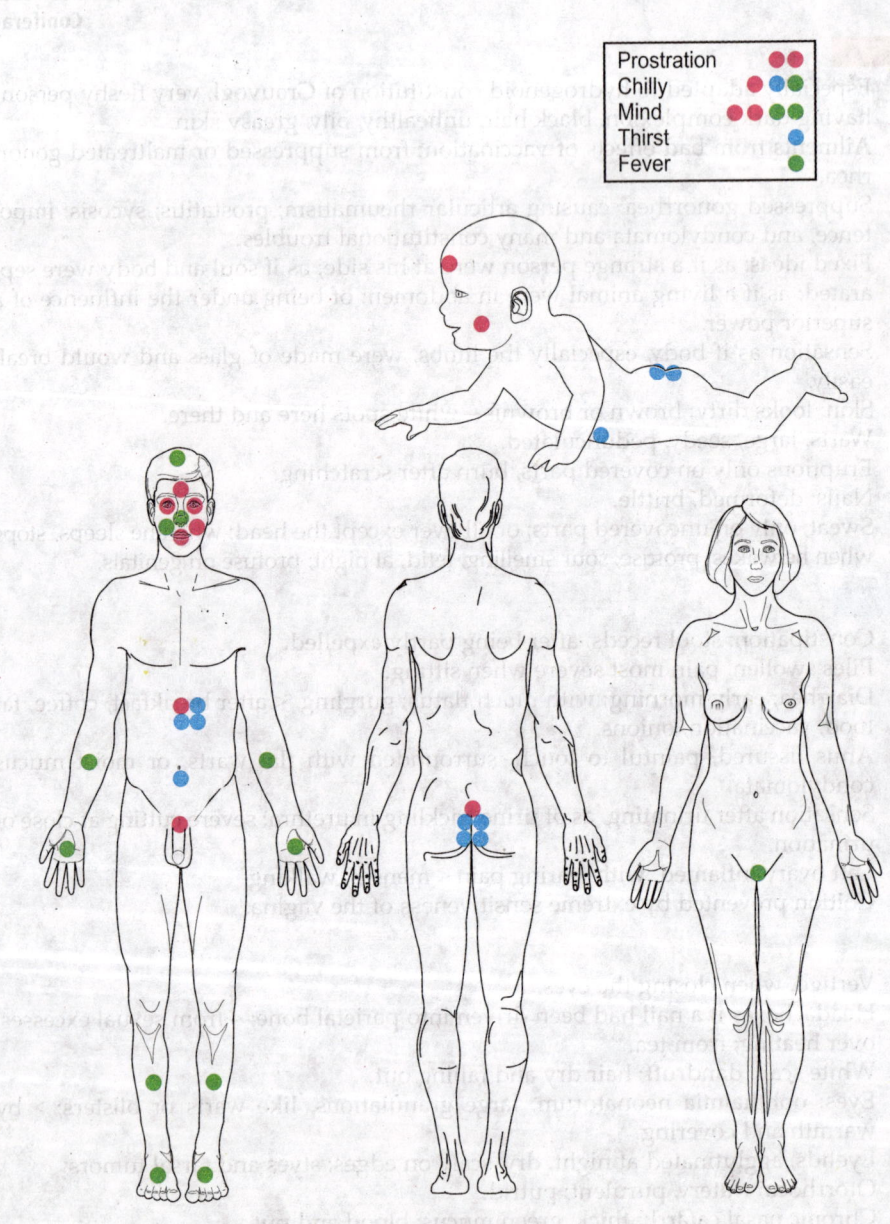

VERATRUM ALBUM

White Hellebore
Melanthaceae

- For children and old people; the extremes of life; young people of a nervous sanguine temperament.
- Adapted to diseases with rapid sinking of the vital forces; complete prostration; collapse.
- Face: pale, blue, collapsed; features sunken, hippocratic; red while lying, becomes pale on rising up.
- Cold perspiration on the forehead; with nearly all complaints.
- Copious evacuations; vomiting, purging; salivation, sweat, urine with profound prostration; coldness; blueness; and collapse.
- Faints from emotions; least exertion; slight injury, with hemorrhage; after stools, vomiting.
- Mania with lewd, lascivious talk, amorous or religious.
- Desire to cut and tear everything, especially clothes.
- Swallows his own excrement.

- Thirst: intense, unquenchable, for large quantities of very cold water.
- Wants everything cold, or sour drinks, juicy fruits and salt.
- Cold feeling in abdomen.
- Violent vomiting with profuse diarrhea.
- Vomiting: excessive with nausea and great prostration; < by drinking; by least motion; great weakness after.
- Diarrhea: frequent, greenish, watery, gushing; mixed with flakes; cutting colic, with cramps in limbs and spreading all over; prostrating.
- Cholera: vomiting and purging; stool, profuse, watery, gushing, prostrating; after fright.
- Constipation: no desire; stool large, hard; in round, black balls; from inactive rectum; painful, of infants and children.

- Sensation of a lump of ice on vertex, with chilliness.
- Icy coldness: of face, tip of nose, feet, legs, hands, arms, and many other parts.
- Dysmenorrhoea with prolapse; with coldness of the body; with vomiting and diarrhea; cold sweat, and fainting with slightest movement.
- In congestive or pernicious intermittent fever, with extreme coldness, thirst, face cold and collapsed.
- Ill effects of fright; disappointed love, injured pride or honor; suppressed exanthema, opium, tobacco, alcohol.